You Can Be Well!

The Five Vital Steps to Wellness

Dr. Stephanie A. Maj

Disclaimer

The information in this book is intended for educational use only and should not be construed as medical advice. You should consult with your physician before attempting any activity or making any lifestyle changes discussed in this book. Although every attempt is made to ensure the accuracy of the information presented, the author and publisher are not liable for any illness or injury that may result from attempting any activities or lifestyle changes presented in this book.

Copper Moon Press
713 Minnehaha Avenue East
St. Paul, MN 55106

The paper used in this publication meets the minimum requirements of the American National Standards for Information Services - Permanence of Paper for Printed Library Materials, ANSI Z39.48-1984.

What People Are Saying About You Can Be Well

"We all need coaches to guide us in new directions. Dr. Stephanie Maj is an incredible Health Coach that can guide you to a new level of health for you and your entire family. Increased health and vitality leads to enhanced wealth and influence. Who wouldn't want more of that! Follow the path and steps that Dr. Maj creates for you in this book and unleash your full potential."

- Dr. Janice Hughes
Founder of 2inspire, www.2inspireonline.com

"Rarely in life are you so incredibly blessed to meet another human being that radiates such love and passion for life. I have been so blessed. Now you are blessed enough to learn from a modern healing master. Allow this book to move you and "You Can Be Well", too."

- C. Bryan Strother, D.C., F.I.C.P.A.
Clinic Director, The Wellness Center

"Dr. Stephanie Maj is a gifted healer, a superb communicator, and a significant contributor to the wellness landscape – pay attention, she will guide you to better health."

- Dr. Dennis Perman
Co-Founder, The Masters Circle

"Your health is your most valuable asset. This book is a wealth of helpful information to guide you to a life of abundant wellness."

- Dr. Jennifer Pitcairn
  Clinic Director, Complete Health Chiropractic Center

"Wellness begins in the heart; if you heal your heart you will heal your body!"

- Michelle Robin, D.C.
  Chief Wellness Officer, Your Wellness Connection, P.A.

"What is the truth to good health? Have you ever wondered? The surprisingly simple answers to this question are contained in this easy to read book by Chicago D.C., Dr. Stephanie Maj. Dr. Maj takes you on a layman's journey through the systems of the body, simple nutrition and simple exercise to empower you to be in charge of the healthy lifestyle you desire and deserve. This is a life-changing book. Enjoy!"

- Catherine McGuire, D.C.
  Monument, CO.

"Your beliefs about what makes you healthy and what steps to take to attain true wellness will become clear with the guidance and wisdom of Dr. Maj. She is a rare warrior willing to stand up and guide us, the people who need her wisdom most. A true blessing!"

- Kari Swain, D.C., D.I.C.C.P.
  Diplomate in Clinical Chiropractic Pediatrics

"This book is a complete guide to living a radiantly healthy, fulfilling life. It is written in an easy to follow format that provides great information without overwhelming detail. For anyone interested in sharing the "Truth" about wellness this easy to read book is a perfect tool. Dr. Maj shares information about the essential components of health with passion, clarity and humor."

- Pat Gayman, D.C.
Authentic Alignment Business Coach
Former Dean of Clinics, Life Chiropractic College West

"Today, people need guidance more than ever about how to care for their bodies to attain health and wellness. Dr. Stephanie Maj has written such a guide. "You Can Be Well" is the perfect instruction manual in taking care of your precious and irreplaceable body, mind and spirit. Everything you need to know about caring for your body is contained in this book! (and it's written by one of my FAVORITE women of all time - my luminous and gifted healer - friend!!)"

- Kristy Taylor, D,C
Klamath Falls, OR

"Clear, precise and direct. Dr. Stephanie Maj has done more for health care than high definition has done for television. Her book is a guide for all who want to achieve wellness. Chicago is blessed to have her in their healthcare community."

- Dr. Marsha K. Heikkinen
Former Vice-Chair, Board of Trustees, Parker College of Chiropractic

Table Of Contents

Acknowledgments

Welcome to the second edition of my book, You Can Be Well! I want to thank all of the people that purchased the first edition of this book. There is nothing better than having someone come to me for help that has already read the book and is "ALL IN!"

So many people come to mind when I think of those I need to thank. This book project started with the inspiration of Dr. Darren Weissman, an amazing healer that started chiropractic school with me back in 1991. His book, "The Power of Infinite Love & Gratitude," spoke to me and was the catalyst for me to begin writing. My healing work with him has opened the door for me to let my vision shine in this book. Many people encouraged me: Marena McPherson, Dr. Patricia Gayman, Dr. Barb Gettel, Dr. Jennifer Pitcairn, Dr. Bryan Strother, and my Royal Chiropractic Knights of the Roundtable. Thank you to my coaches Dr. Pat Gayman and Dr. Janice Hughes, two amazing women who live with integrity and purpose and who I would love to be like when I grow up!

I want to send a shout out to my family, especially my many nieces and nephews. You all give me the reason to want to make this world a better place. It is my desire to show up as the best me possible so that I can be an example to all of you that you can do anything in life, even change the world. I promised I would mention them all by name: Sam, Sarah, Becca, Kayla, Cody, Shelby, Mackenzie, Megan, and Olivia. I love you all.

I have to acknowledge my amazing staff. I believe my clinic has the best patients and the best staff ever. They get the big picture that it is not about us; it is about delivering great service and not getting in the way of the healing process.

Lastly, I would like to thank Julie Heator, my editor, proofreader, partner, wife and best friend. Without your support, none of this dream life could be possible. Thank you.

The Five Vital Steps to Health and Wellness

The tagline in my office is "Community Chiropractic: A Journey to Health and Wellness!" To talk about the journey to health we must first discuss the journey to sickness. The journey to sickness is often considered an event. What that means is everyday a patient will ask me, "What do you think I did doc?" They want to know what ONE thing caused the state of their health. It wasn't the box you lifted, the sock you tried to pick up a minute before your back when out, or the bug going around your office.

The state of your health or lack thereof is a process—a process of many, many different factors combining over time to get you to the place you are with regard to your health. It takes us lots of time to gain the weight yet we are all looking for the quick fix to take it off. There are no quick fixes in the weight loss arena and there are no quick fixes when it comes to your journey back to health. Every fall I write my flu shot article in my newsletter. The crux is that it is appealing to think that just getting this shot will ensure you will not be sick that winter. You can eat, drink and smoke to excess and that shot will protect you. Unfortunately it doesn't work that way.

Health is a journey, a process as well. I have condensed this process into the 5 Vital Steps to Health and Wellness. They are:

1. Remove Nerve Interference
2. Achieve an Ideal Weight
3. Beat Stress
4. Exercise as a Nutrient
5. Eliminate Toxins

Understanding how our bodies work is vital on the road back to wellness. Let's dive in and explain in detail some factors necessary for health.

Why I Wrote This Book

It is not an accident you picked up this book. I want you to know that if you read and absorb the ideas and actions in this book you can live the promise, "You Can Be Well!" This is a textbook to a healthier life. Like any textbook, there is some theory and lots of action and exercises to perform. You can read this book like a novel, letting the words wash over you and saying to yourself, "I know that." My question to you is this: knowing it and living it are two different things. I challenge you to dig into this book, ask yourself which areas of your body and your life you have been ignoring and need to heal.

My name is Dr. Stephanie Maj. I am a Chiropractor. I am an author. Welcome to the second edition of my book. I am going to tell you the story of why I wrote this book but first I want to explain why I am writing a second edition. The first edition of the book needed to be changed a bit to help people navigate where to best direct their attention when it comes to improving their health. "5 Vital Steps to Health and Wellness" was born out of my using this book in my office to coach people back to health. Vital steps, because like your vital signs, they are necessary for life.

Also, I feel strongly that I missed something BIG in my first edition...Achieving an Ideal Weight. Every year the statistics come out that Americans are getting fatter and fatter. Obesity is the #1 preventable cause of disease, overtaking smoking. I have devoted an entire step to the goal of achieving an ideal weight.

Now on to my story…how I became a Chiropractor is not all that exciting and yet it's my story and I am going to tell it here. I got injured, had spinal pain and my mom urged me to go to a Chiropractor. She also urged me to be a Chiropractor. "Chiropractor?" There are none in our family and to my knowledge no one in my family had ever been adjusted.

So I went to Dr. Tony Battaglia in my hometown of Akron, Ohio. I was 23 years old working in an environmental lab and I felt lost. I hated my job and I was looking for deeper meaning in my life. I went to his office looking for pain relief and received so much more. I was assigned a young doctor, excited and passionate about what he did and how he was going to help lots of people. No one talked about helping people at my lab job. Intrigued, I dug deeper.

From my earliest memory, I had always wanted to be a doctor. A pediatrician to be exact. Through my undergraduate studies at Ohio University, I was a Nutrition premed major and just assumed my path was to be a medical doctor. After going through the application process I realized that there was something that didn't fit about me and traditional medicine. I decided against that career for reasons that were not fully formed in my mind and have since become crystal clear to me.

After completing my treatment plan with my Chiropractor, my sprained neck healed AND my lifelong headaches went away as well. I decided that I needed to get my life moving in a better direction so off I went to Chiropractic school in Chicago. Chiropractic school is a 5 year program, where we study the biomechanics, neurology, and function of the body more extensively than medical school students. I spent my last year and a half of school in clinics, helping the community and firming up my techniques of diagnosis and treatment.

School was the most intense experience of my life. It was hard to think of life after school and the direction of my new career. I just wanted to help people, that's all. I saw that there were so many people to help; this world has never been sicker. I felt that working under another Chiropractor for a time was important. In that experience I learned many things both clinical and business. My biggest lesson was that I could make a living, help lots of people, and do it with integrity and honesty.

I opened Community Chiropractic in Chicago on April 1, 1996, my 30th birthday. The first years are a blur. Keeping a business open is a struggle the first couple years in any endeavor. I never doubted I would succeed. There were lots of people that were there in those early days that are still around today. I was truly 'practicing' on them and I am grateful for their loyalty.

My patient base at the time consisted mostly of the usual neck and back pain patients plus lots of headache sufferers. I feel strongly in the value of Chiropractic in caring and curing people of those debilitating conditions. I am amazed everyday when someone who comes to the clinic gets significant relief of a longstanding condition in a short time. They always exclaim,

"Why didn't my medical doctor tell me about Chiropractic instead of giving me all the drugs and surgeries?" My answer is simple, "Does Pepsi tell you to drink Coke?"

It was this divide that has driven me to step out into the forefront of the Wellness Movement. What does that mean? Well...wellness is a lifestyle. This means it is the result of healthy actions taken in a consistent manner. It is not an event, a one shot deal, a little purple pill. They will never find the cure to most cancers and diseases because most are the result of a toxic and deficient life. Most people are taught they are a victim of their health. Not so. How do most people unknowingly and knowingly set the ball rolling toward illness? What was that process and how can it be arrested and reversed? Who is going to coach people to live more in line with natural laws? Who will lead people to the path of health and wellness? That is my mission. That is my purpose. That is what this book is about.

After many years in practice, I had had enough. If people knew what I knew, they would do what I do. I had to step out of my comfort zone. I had to start speaking to others about what health really is and what it will take to get you there. That is when I obtained a certification in Pediatrics and Prenatal care. I can't just help sick adults when most of them started out as sick kids. I have to teach young parents how to grow healthy families. Every parent's hope is that their kids have more than they did. Well, the last thing kids need is more stuff. They need to know how their bodies work and more education on what will make them well. No one taught me that as a kid. That is why I wrote this book.

I have to use my pickle analogy. How do you make a pickle? Well, you stick a cucumber into brine and eventually it turns into a pickle. At some early points in the process, you could take it out and it would still be a cucumber, right? At some point though, that cucumber turns into a pickle and there is NOTHING you can do to turn it back. It's a pickle now. Our health is the same way. Early in our lives we are that cucumber and just take for granted that we will always have our health. We spend little time, effort and money to make sure we stay well. Then it happens like it happens to so many people. We turn into that pickle. We get sick and our health starts slipping from us. It is at this time that all our time, effort and money goes to trying in vain to change this sick pickle body back to the cucumber. We all know of someone who has flown all over the globe to find an experimental cure to their life threatening disease. Most 'cures' unfortunately don't work. I want to get to you before you are a pickle, while we still have a chance to turn this whole thing around. That is why I wrote this book.

The World Health Organization defines health as "a state of complete physical, mental, and social well-being, not merely the absence of disease or infirmity." Health is not merely the absence of disease any more than wealth is an absence of poverty. Health is not simply 'feeling fine,' for we know that problems may progress for years without causing any symptoms whatsoever, such as heart disease and cancer.

The key to health is to become a proactive agent for your body and not wait until you hurt before you do something about your health. The answer is not to spend more money on expensive medical tests or procedures, or to consume more prescription drugs, but rather to change how we think about health and disease.

In the dizzying array of choices in health care today, it is sometimes hard to know what to believe or what to think. New and very expensive medical tests and procedures are introduced each year that do very little to improve health. Revolutionary diet and exercise programs emerge on an almost daily basis promising health and happiness. Carefully crafted pharmaceutical ads show how happy you could be if you simply took this drug or that drug. Do you realize that the United States has only 5% of the world's population, yet we consume almost half of the world's supply of prescription drugs? You would think that if drugs were the answer to health that we would have the healthiest nation in the world. But, unfortunately, that is not the case. In fact, the general population is getting heavier, the rates of diabetes, heart disease and cancer are rapidly rising, and we have one of the highest infant mortality rates in the civilized world – behind the entire European Union as well as countries like Cuba, South Korea, Singapore, Aruba, Greece and the Czech Republic.

Today more than ever, tens of millions of Americans are seeking alternative opinions on how to treat and prevent disease. What accounts for this major paradigm shift? Orthodox medicine has not lived up to its billing as the be-all and end-all in health care. Traditional medicine does some great things, don't get me wrong, especially when it comes to treating life-threatening trauma and surgical repair of damaged body parts. But when it comes to the management of the chronic degenerative conditions that affect most people, traditional medicine falls short.

One reason for this is that traditional medicine does not focus its attention on the prevention of disease. Rather, its focus is on trying to treat disease once it occurs. It focuses on the pickles, paying little or no attention to the cucumber. Health insurance is the same way. It is not health care but sick care. It could just as easily be called Pickle Care!

Most people in Western civilization have become high stress, fast paced and toxic. We have lost step with nature. We eat unnatural foods, don't get enough exercise, are overweight and when our body begins to break down, we attempt to manage it through numerous prescription drugs.

As a Chiropractor, I take a very different approach than that taken by medical doctors. I teach people that it is much better to prevent disease from happening in the first place than to try to treat it once it occurs. By creating a state of optimal health within your body, you will feel better, have more energy, and an increased quality of life. You will also avoid the expense and pain associated with getting hooked into the downward spiral of disease and dependence on more and more prescription medications.

Chiropractors are more than just ache and pain doctors. Chiropractic is based on the concept that within every living thing there is an inborn, innate wisdom always striving for radiant health. The body has a tremendous capacity to heal itself if it is allowed to do so. My job is simply to identify and remove the obstacles that prevent the body from being healthy. To accomplish this, I employ a variety of physical therapies such as chiropractic adjustments, trigger point therapy, stretches, exercises and other lifestyle changes.

None of this information is new to my patients; they hear me teach this in my clinic every day. The problem is that if you are not in my clinic, you miss out. Second, my hope is that this book can serve to help all of the people out there who suffer needlessly, simply because they don't understand what Chiropractic is and how it can help them. This also includes many medical doctors who still buy into the common myths surrounding Chiropractic care, such as the myth that Chiropractic adjustments are dangerous. In fact, you are thousands of times more likely to suffer a negative reaction from taking an aspirin than from getting a Chiropractic adjustment. Third, and most important, I am writing this book to inspire you to live the truth that You Can Be Well, and live a radiantly healthy life, free from pain and disease.

Picking up this book was no accident. You Can Be Well! Let me help you on your journey to health and wellness.

1

Vital Step One: Remove Nerve Interference

As a chiropractor, this is by far my favorite chapter. This chapter encompasses the core ideas in this book. The biggest misconception about Chiropractic is that it is about the spine. Yes, as a doctor of Chiropractic, I am interested in the spine because the nerves come out in between each of those vertebrae. Lack of proper alignment (subluxation is the chiropractic word for that) interferes with those nerves and interferes with the normal function of the body.

The results of a poorly functioning nerve system can be devastating. Lack of proper alignment chokes off the normal flow of the body and sends all the systems into crisis mode. One of the most common things I hear on a daily basis is that I don't think I am sick yet I don't feel well. This is the plight of many in my community. I am here to tell you that NO DRUG is going to fix this!

Core Ideas in Vital Step One: Removing Nerve Interference

- *The body is a self-healing, self-regulating organism;*
- *The nervous system is the master controller of all these systems;*
- *Interference in the body's nervous system by subluxation interferes with the body's ability to heal and function properly;*
- *Chiropractic removes the interference caused by subluxation and restores the body's ability to repair and regulate its systems.*

What is Health?

According to the World Health Organization, "Health is a state of complete physical, mental, and social well-being, not merely the absence of disease or sickness." Disease could be present in your body right now, but you're unaware of it because you are not experiencing any symptoms. For example, research reveals that coronary heart disease is the leading killer of Americans (Framingham Heart Study NHLBI). But in fact, 57% of men who died suddenly from coronary heart disease had NO previous symptoms of the disease.

Normal function is imperative to having a healthy body. The key to health is function. That is why it is important to know your body is functioning by having it checked by a chiropractor. Chiropractors increase the function of your body by removing the interference in nerves.

Feelings vs. Function

One of the biggest misconceptions is that you can feel your level of health. Many health problems occur without symptoms, including cancer, diabetes, and heart disease.

The nervous system is made up of trillions of highly-specialized individual nerve cells, each of which communicate with hundreds or thousands of other nerve cells through tiny electrical pulses. The nervous system is called the master controller as it is responsible for the control of all major body functions including our senses, movement and balance, as well as the regulations of all body functions. Most people only think of pain when they think of their nerves, yet pain nerves consist of only 5-8% of the entire nervous system.

Vertebral Subluxation: The Enemy of Health

Vertebral subluxation (misalignment) is an enemy of the central nervous system. Various stresses can cause misaligned vertebrae, known as subluxation, which disturbs the communication within the nervous system, resulting in abnormal function. Physical, chemical and mental/emotional stresses are the main causes of subluxations and cause your quality of health to decline whether or not symptoms are present.

This is similar to a car's wheels being out of alignment, which causes the tires to wear out faster than normal. Driving on a worn tire puts the driver at risk of a blowout, possibly leading to costly damage and increasing the potential for an accident. For any problem, the increase in time the problem has been present increases the risk.

What truly differentiates doctors of chiropractic from any other healthcare professionals is the fact that chiropractors are the only doctors who are trained to diagnose and treat what are called spinal subluxations. Like dentists look for cavities (tooth decay), chiropractors look for subluxation (the beginning of spinal decay). The word "subluxation" comes from the Latin words meaning "to dislocate" (luxare) and "somewhat or slightly" (sub). So the term 'vertebral subluxation' literally means a slight dislocation (misalignment) of the bones in the spine.

Although this term was adequate in the 1800s when much was still misunderstood about the human body, today the word "subluxation" has changed in meaning to capture the complex of neurological, structural and functional changes that occur when a bone is "out of place." For this reason chiropractors usually refer to subluxations of the spine as the "Vertebral Subluxation Complex", or "VSC" for short. There are actually five components that contribute to the vertebral subluxation complex (VSC). They are:

The Bone Component

The vertebrae are either out of position, not moving properly, or are undergoing degeneration. This frequently leads to a narrowing of the spaces between the bones through which the nerves pass; often resulting in irritation or impingement of the nerve itself.

The Nervous Component

The disruption of the normal flow of energy along the nerve fibers, causing the messages traveling along the nerves to become distorted. The result is that all of the tissues that are fed by those nerves receive distorted signals from the brain and, consequently, are not able to function normally. Over time, this can lead to a whole host of conditions, such as peptic ulcers, constipation and other organ system dysfunction.

The muscular component. Since nerves control the muscles that help hold the vertebrae in place, muscles have to be considered to be an integral part of the vertebral subluxation complex. In fact, muscles both affect, and are affected by the VSC. A subluxation can irritate a nerve, the irritated nerve can cause a muscle to spasm, the spasmed muscle pulls the attached vertebrae further out of place, which then further irritates the nerve and you have a vicious cycle. It is no wonder that very few subluxations just go away by themselves.

The soft tissue component. The VSC will also affect the surrounding tendons, ligaments, blood supply, and other tissues as the misaligned vertebrae tug and squeeze the connective tissue with tremendous force. Over time, the soft tissues can become stretched out or scarred, leaving the spine with either a permanent instability or restriction.

Your Nervous System

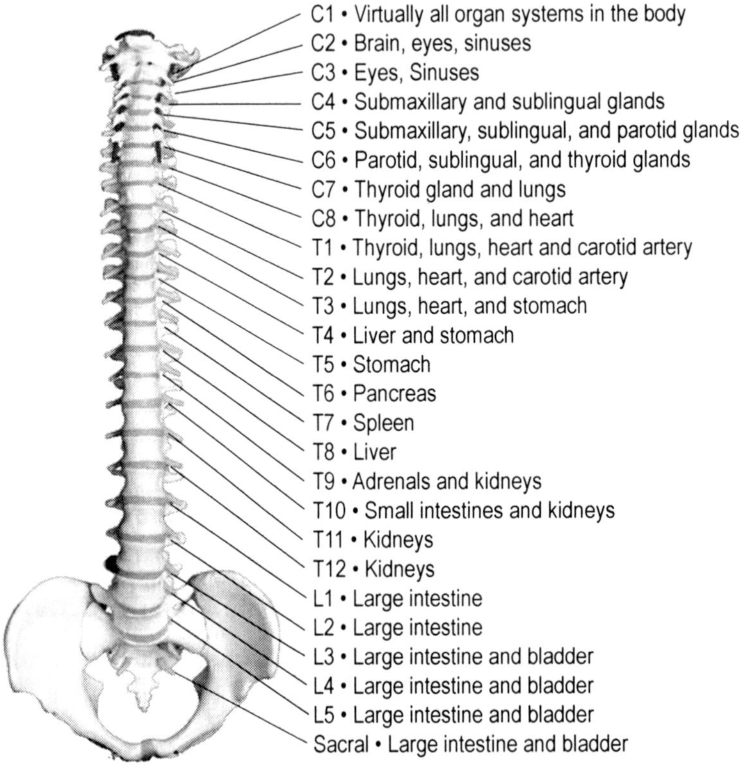

All of the functions related to the human body are controlled by the extensive neural network continually sending and receiving electrical impulses to and from the brain. Stress in any part of the nervous system may result in a variety of health problems throughout the body.

The Chemical Component

This is the change in the chemistry of the body due to the VSC. Most often, the chemical changes, such as the release of a class of chemicals called "kinins," are pro-inflammatory; meaning that they increase inflammation in the affected area.

When subluxation is present, it starts a major chain of events. This neural cascade causes muscle injury, stress hormone release, decrease in the immune system, increases in blood pressure, and an overall strain on the bodily systems.

More and more scientific research is demonstrating the tremendous detrimental impact that subluxations have on the tissue of the body. In order to be truly healthy, it is vital that your nervous system be functioning free of interference from subluxations. Chiropractors are the only health professionals trained in the detection, location, and correction of the vertebral subluxation complex through the chiropractic adjustment.

Chiropractic
The Best Kept Secret in Health Care

The word "chiropractic" comes from the Greek words cheir (hand) and praxis (action) and literally means "done by hand." Instead of prescribing drugs or performing surgeries, chiropractors use manual treatments of the spine and joints, exercise therapy, massage, trigger point therapy and lifestyle changes to allow the body's natural state of health to fully express itself.

Like conventional medicine, chiropractic is based upon scientific principles of (1) diagnosis through testing and empirical observation and (2) treatment based upon the practitioner's rigorous training and clinical experience. But unlike conventional medicine, which focuses on attempting to treat disease once it occurs, chiropractic attempts to improve the health of the individual in an effort to avoid illness in the first place. Most people would rather be healthy and avoid illness if they could. This is one of the main reasons for the big upsurge in the popularity of chiropractic. People are recognizing the benefit of seeking an alternative to traditional medicine; one that will help them achieve and maintain optimal health.

We understand that one of the main causes of pain and disease is the misalignment and abnormal motion of the vertebrae in the spinal column called a subluxation. Chiropractic works by removing these subluxations in the spine, thereby relieving pressure and irritation on the nerves, restoring joint mobility, and returning the body back to a state of normal function.

Numerous studies have demonstrated that chiropractic care is one of the most effective treatments for back pain, neck pain, headaches, whiplash, sports injuries and many other types of musculoskeletal problems. It has even been shown to be effective in reducing high blood pressure, decreasing the frequency of childhood ear infections (otitis media) and improving the symptoms of asthma.

The chiropractic approach to healthcare is holistic, meaning that it addresses your overall health. I recognize that many lifestyle factors such as exercise, diet, rest and your environment impact your health. For this reason, I recommend changes in lifestyle— eating, exercise, and sleeping habits—in addition to chiropractic care.

What is Chiropractic Care?

Spinal adjustments to correct subluxations are what make doctors of chiropractic unique in comparison with any other type of health care professional. The term "adjustment" refers to the specific manipulation chiropractors apply to vertebrae that have abnormal movement patterns or fail to function normally. The objective of the chiropractic treatment is to reduce the subluxation, which results in an increased range of motion, reduced nerve irritability and improved function.

Chiropractic is so much more than simply a means of relieving pain. Ultimately, the goal of the chiropractic treatment is to restore the body to its natural state of optimal health. In order to accomplish this, I use a variety of treatment methods, including manual adjustments, Pro-Adjuster® adjustments, acupuncture, trigger point therapy, nutrition, exercise rehabilitation, massage, as well as counseling on lifestyle issues that impact your health. Since the body has a remarkable ability to heal itself and to maintain its own health, my primary focus is simply to remove those things which interfere with the body's normal healing ability.

Chiropractors understand that within each of us is an innate wisdom, a health energy that will express itself as perfect health and well-being if we simply allow it to. Therefore, the focus of chiropractic care is simply to remove any physiological blocks to the proper expression of the body's innate wisdom. Once these subluxations are removed, health is the natural result.

Manual Manipulation

Manual manipulations of the spine and other joints in the body have been around for a long time. Ancient writings from China and Greece dating between 2700 B.C. and 1500 B.C. mention spinal manipulation and the maneuvering of the lower extremities to ease low back pain. In fact, Hippocrates, the famous Greek physician who lived from 460 to 357 B.C., published a text detailing the importance of manual manipulation. In one of his writings he declares, "Get knowledge of the spine, for this is the requisite for many diseases."

Evidence of manual manipulation of the body has been found among the ancient civilizations of Egypt, Babylon, Syria, Japan, the Incas, Mayans and Native Americans. The understanding of the human frame or structure and its relationship to human function or health has been around since ancient times and is best described by the famous Thomas Edison quote: "The doctor of the future will give no medicine, but will interest his patients in the care of the human frame, in diet, and in the cause and prevention of disease."

Pro-Adjuster: A Breakthrough in Healing

Imagine thirty or forty years ago, if I told you that dentistry would be painless, that doctors would watch television to perform surgeries, that brain surgery for tumors could be done with a laser, that fetuses could be operated on within the uterus, that knife-less surgery could be performed, you would not have believed me. By the same token, would you believe me if I told you that chiropractic adjustments could be done painlessly without any popping or cracking sounds, and no jerking or pulling of the body and neck? Would you believe that newborns as well as the elderly with osteoporosis could be treated effortlessly?

The facts are that all these high tech procedures were once just a dream in someone's head and now are reality and commonplace. The future is now! Advances in computers and engineering technology have been able to uniquely blend chiropractic in order to both analyze and care for the human body in such a way that was never before realized. This advancement is a new technology called the Pro-Adjuster®. The Pro-Adjuster® is the most advanced computerized method of chiropractic care that exists in our profession today.

Chiropractors and their patients know that manual adjustments are safe and effective, regardless of what technique is used, as long as the doctor has the knowledge and skill to apply the method properly. However, sometimes people who have never experienced a chiropractic adjustment may be fearful because of something they have seen, read or been told about what they might see, feel, or experience with a chiropractic adjustment.

Occasionally people have a fear of the unfamiliar. With the use of the Pro-Adjuster® equipment and techniques, virtually all of these fears simply disappear. If you are looking for the perfect spinal adjustment—one that is precise, painless, and effective, without popping or cracking noises—then the Pro-Adjuster® is the ideal solution for you.

The amount of force (pressure) that the Pro-Adjuster® uses to make an adjustment of your spine is an amount equivalent to tapping your fingers on a table. Let's test this out. Put your hand flat on a table or even your leg. Now tap your fingers as though you were listening to music that you really enjoyed. Now tap as hard as you can. That is about the amount of pressure you will feel with a Pro-Adjuster® adjustment. Do you think you can handle that? Of course you can. Even small children are adjusted with the Pro-Adjuster®. The amount of pressure can be completely controlled and adjusted for the patient's comfort, safety and effectiveness.

How can anything so gentle with such little force involved move my vertebrae and change my spine? The Pro-Adjuster® utilizes a precise oscillating force with uninterrupted motion. It is able to increase the mobility of the spinal vertebrae by reducing or eliminating the fixations. In other words, the Pro-Adjuster® is "unsticking" the joint.

Have you ever seen a woodpecker tapping in an oscillating fashion on a tree? It is hard to believe, but you can watch them bore right through the hardest wood! The Pro-Adjuster® taps in much the same way but uses soft tips that are comfortable to the human body and don't create damage.

Not only is the Pro-Adjuster® great for the patient, it is great for the doctors as well. It is a valuable tool providing vital information about your spinal health, ultimately resulting in a higher level of care. What is it that every doctor wants for their patient and what every patient wants from their doctor? The answer is one word...RESULTS! The more the doctor knows about the patient, the better the result. The more a patient knows and understands about their condition, the better their results will be.

The Three Phases of Chiropractic Care

Chiropractic care following an injury is like building a house – certain things have to happen in a particular sequence in order for everything to stand strong and work the way it is supposed to. If you tried to put up your walls before you had a solid foundation, your walls would be weak and eventually collapse. If you tried to put on your roof before the walls were ready, you would run into the same problem. The same is true for your body. Your body has to go through a particular plan of care in order to repair itself correctly and fully. There are three general phases of chiropractic care; 1) relief care, 2) corrective care, and, 3) wellness.

Phase One - Relief Care

Some people go to a chiropractor because they are in pain. In this first phase of care, the main goal is to relieve you of your symptoms. Sometimes this will require daily visits, or three to four times a week for an initial series of visits—the number of visits per week depends on the severity of your condition.

Most people are under the assumption that if they don't feel any pain that there is nothing wrong with them – that they are healthy. Unfortunately, pain is a very poor indicator of health. In fact, pain and other symptoms frequently only appear after a disease or other condition has become advanced. For example, consider a cavity in your tooth. Does it hurt when it first develops or after it has become serious? How about heart disease? Do you realize that the first symptom that many people with heart disease experience is a heart attack? Regardless of whether you are talking about cancer, heart disease, diabetes, stress or problems with the spine, pain is usually the last thing to appear. When you begin chiropractic care, pain is also the first symptom to disappear, even though much of the underlying condition remains.

Phase Two – Corrective/Restorative Care

Most chiropractors regard the elimination of symptoms as the easiest part of a person's care. If all that the chiropractor does is to remove the pain and stop there, the chances of the condition recurring are much greater. In order to avoid a rapid recurrence of symptoms, it is necessary to continue care even though your symptoms are gone.

During the correction/restorative phase of care, you will not have to receive adjustments as often as you did during the

The Three Phases of Chiropractic Care		
Phase 1	Phase 2	Phase 3
Acute Care The first objective is to help you feel better. During this phase, the goal is to relieve pain.	**Stabilization** During the corrective care phase, muscles and other tissues are allowed to heal more completely, thereby helping to prevent re-injury.	**Wellness Care** Once your body has fully healed, it is important to come in for periodic adjustments to improve your well-being.

first phase of care and, depending on your particular circumstances, may begin doing exercises and stretches at home to help accelerate your healing. Do not be discouraged if you have mild flare-ups in your symptoms on occasion. This is normal. Flare-ups are bound to occur during the corrective phase because your body has not fully recovered. Depending on the severity of your injury or condition and how long you have been suffering from it, this phase of your care may last anywhere from a few months to a couple of years.

Phase Three - Wellness Care

Once your body has fully healed, routine wellness chiropractic care can help to ensure that your physical problems do not return and keep your body in optimal condition. Just like continuing an exercise program and eating well in order to sustain the benefits of exercise and proper diet, it is necessary to continue chiropractic care to ensure the health of your musculo-skeletal system. When you make routine chiropractic care a part of your lifestyle, you avoid many of the aches and pains that so many people suffer though, your joints will last longer and you will be able to engage in more of the activities you love. Spinal misalignments are much like diabetes, in that you can't just treat it once and expect everything to be better. It requires that you take care of yourself on a regular basis to remain healthy. Just like with diabetes, if you neglect to take care of your spine, over time your health will suffer – usually without any symptoms—until the problems have become severe. This is why I often call spinal subluxations "diabetes of the spine." It's not that your spine has diabetes, but rather to drive home

The Myths and Facts about Chiropractic

As successful as chiropractic has become, there are a lot of myths about chiropractic floating around in the general public. Times have definitely changed for the better, but the fact is that many people still do not understand what chiropractors do. Let's talk about a few of the more common myths about chiropractic.

Myth #1 - Chiropractors are not real doctors

Chiropractors are licensed as health care providers in every U.S. state and most of countries around the world. While the competition to attend chiropractic school is not as fierce as medical school, the chiropractic and medical school curricula are virtually identical. In fact, chiropractors have more hours of education than their medical counterparts. As part of their education, chiropractic students also complete approximately nine hundred hours of work in a clinical setting assisting licensed chiropractors. Once chiropractic students graduate, they have to pass four sets of national board exams as well as state board exams in the states they want to practice.

Chiropractors receive extensive training, combined with many hours of practical work. Just like conventional medical doctors, chiropractors are medical professionals that are subject to the same testing, licensing and monitoring by state and national peer-reviewed boards. Federal and state programs, such as Medicare, Medicaid and Workers' Compensations programs cover chiropractic, and all federal agencies accept sick-leave certificates signed by doctors of chiropractic.

The biggest difference between chiropractors and medical doctors lies not in their education or diagnostic ability, but in their preferred method of treatment. Medical doctors are trained in the use of medicines (chemicals that affect your internal biochemistry) and surgery. Consequently, if you have a chemical problem, such as diabetes, hypothyroid or an infection, medical doctors can be very helpful.

However, if your problem is that one of the bones in your spine is out of place, or you have trigger points in your muscles that are causing pain, there is no drug in existence that can fix it. You need a physical treatment to correct a physical problem. That's where chiropractic really shines. Chiropractors use physical treatments—adjustments, exercises, stretches, muscle therapy—to treat conditions that are physical, rather than chemical, in origin; such as back pain, muscle spasms, headaches, poor posture, etc.

Myth #2 - Medical doctors don't like chiropractors

The American Medical Association's opposition to chiropractic was at its strongest in the 1940s under the leadership of Morris Fishbein. Fishbein called chiropractors "rabid dogs" and referred to them as "playful and cute, but killers." He tried to portray chiropractors as members of an unscientific cult, caring about nothing but taking their patients money. Up to the late 1970s and early 1980s, the medical establishment purposely conspired to try to destroy the profession of chiropractic. In fact, in a landmark lawsuit in the 1980s found that the American Medical Association was guilty of conspiracy and was ordered to pay restitution to the American Chiropractic Association.

In the 20 years since, the position of most medical doctors has changed; mostly because of several major studies that showed the superiority of chiropractic in treating a host of conditions, coupled with a better understanding among medical doctors about what chiropractors actually do. Many hospitals across the country now have chiropractors on staff and many chiropractic offices have medical doctors on staff.

Chiropractors and medical doctors are now much more comfortable working together in cases where medical care is necessary as an adjunct to chiropractic care.

Myth #3 - Once you start going to a chiropractor, you have to keep going the rest of your life

This is a statement that I frequently hear when the topic of chiropractic care comes up in conversation. This statement is only partly true. You only have to continue going to the chiropractor as long as you wish to maintain the health of your neuromusculoskeletal system. Going to a chiropractor is much like going to the dentist, exercising at a gym or eating a healthier diet, as long as you keep it up, you continue to enjoy the benefits.

Many years ago, dentists convinced everyone that the best time to go to the dentist is before your teeth hurt – that routine dental care will help your teeth remain healthy for a long time. It is important to remember that, just like your teeth, your spine experiences normal wear and tear – you walk, drive, sit, lift, sleep and bend. Regular chiropractic care can help you feel better, move with more freedom, and stay healthier throughout your lifetime. Although you can enjoy the benefits of chiropractic care even if you are only treated for a short time, the real benefits come into play when you make chiropractic care a part of your lifestyle.

Myth #4 - Chiropractic adjustments will cause you to have a stroke

Strokes are definitely a serious event, no doubt, and there are some medical doctors who still tell their patients to avoid going to the chiropractor because sooner or later, they say, adjustments of the neck will cause a stroke. There is no denying that a possibility of this happening exists. However, the risk of suffering a stroke from a chiropractic adjustment is extremely small; about the risk of being struck by lightning. In fact, you are 70,000 times more likely to suffer a stroke from the daily use of aspirin to prevent heart attacks than to suffer a stroke from a chiropractic adjustment. You are 37,000 times more likely to suffer a stroke for some unknown reason than to suffer a stroke from a chiropractic adjustment. When administered by a licensed doctor of chiropractic, adjustments are extremely safe.

Frequently Asked Questions

Q. How can I tell if I need to see a chiropractor?

There are several ways you can test yourself and family members to determine whether you should go to a chiropractor for evaluation:

- *Check your posture in a mirror. Remember, posture is a window to your spine. If you see one shoulder higher, your head tilts, one of your hips is higher than the other; this is often an indicator that you are misaligned.*

- *Lie face down and ask someone to look at your heels and see if they are even. If one leg is contracted or shorter than the other, this often means you are misaligned.*
- *Feel your neck and shoulders. Do the muscles feel relaxed or at ease? Compare the muscle tone of your neck and shoulders to the tone of your bicep when it is relaxed. If your neck and shoulders feel tense, you likely have unnec- essary spinal stress.*
- *Turn your head to the right and then left. Do they turn equally as far? Does one side appear tighter than the other? Ask someone to watch you to see whether you can turn more to one side than the other.*

Other indications that you may need to see a chiropractor to get your spine checked:

- *Hearing sounds in your neck or back when you move.*
- *Uneven wearing on the heels of your shoes.*
- *One of your feet flares when you walk.*
- *Aches and pains in your head, neck, shoulders, arms, mid-back, low back or down your legs.*

If you are unsure, I recommend you go to a chiropractor for an initial evaluation and let them give you their professional opinion about your alignment. The truth is most people go through their whole lives never having their spine checked.

When is the best time to realign your spine, when the problem has severely progressed or early on before permanent damage occurs?

Q. What should I expect at my chiropractic appointment?

Consultation

On your first visit to the office you will be welcomed and given a brief tour of the clinic. You first visit is designed for the doctor to learn about you, your condition, and your expectations to determine whether chiropractic care will help you meet your goals. Wellness chiropractors will ask you questions about your lifestyle habits and personal goals.

Examination

After your consultation, you will have an examination. This may include testing your reflexes, your ability to turn and bend as well as other standard chiropractic, orthopedic, neurologic, postural, and physical examinations. Our doctors use advanced technologies to better understand your condition such as surface EMG, thermography, digital foot scans, bio-impedance analysis and electronic meridian testing. If necessary, x-rays may be taken to get a more in-depth look at your spine.

X-rays

X-rays are sometimes required to get a full evaluation of a client. The need for x-rays is considered on a case by case basis. X-rays are very valuable to actually visualize your spine. No one would think of letting a dentist fill a cavity without an x-ray of the tooth. X-rays provide a deeper look that allows doctors to get patients better quicker. Most people are amazed once they see their x-rays and can often immediately identify their misalignments and degeneration.

Report of Findings

Once all the information and examinations have been performed, the doctor will give you a report of findings and answer these four most popular questions:

1) Can you help me?
2) What do you recommend that I do to get better?
3) How long will it take to get well?
4) How much is this going to cost?

Often the report of findings is done on the second visit in order to allow the doctor sufficient time to develop the x-rays and analyze to test results to come up with the most effective course of treatment. If the doctor believes chiropractic care can help you, she will recommend a course of care. Sometimes recommendation for products such as special pillows, supplements or orthotics will accelerate the healing process.

Receiving Care

Most people begin to experience benefits from the very first adjustment. The adjustment is interactive, so you can express any concerns you have and discover the style of adjustment you will be most comfortable with: Pro-Adjuster® or a more manual approach.

Q. What is a chiropractic adjustment?

The chiropractic adjustment is a gentle, quick thrust to a particular joint, typically in the spine, intended to restore normal position and movement. Adjustments can be performed by hand in a manual approach or with the Pro-Adjuster® equipment. Adjustments are important for releasing adhesions in the joint and reducing stress on the nervous system. Because of the fact that the nervous system is that master controller of all muscles and organs in the body, removing stress on the nervous system through chiropractic adjustments will frequently lead to improved health in the entire body.

Q. How many adjustments will I need?

The total number of adjustments you need depends on five main factors: 1) your age, 2) your overall health, 3) the severity of your condition, 4) how long you have had your condition, and 5) what your ultimate goals are. If you are young, in good health and have a mild condition that occurred very recently, you will need far fewer adjustments than if you are older, in poor general health and have been struggling with a problem for many years. The total number of adjustments you will need also depends on whether you are just interested in reducing the pain you are currently experiencing, or are interested in creating optimal long-term health.

Q. Will adjustments hurt?

Usually not. There have been some patients of mine who have experienced mild soreness after being adjusted, but this is more of the exception. Most people feel better very quickly after being adjusted.

Q. Will there be side effects?

Patients may or may not experience side effects from chiropractic treatment. Effects may include temporary discomfort in parts of the body that were treated, headache, or tiredness. These effects tend to be minor and to resolve within 1 to 2 days.

Q. Do I still need to see the chiropractor if my pain is gone?

It is very common for pain to disappear long before the total correction of your condition is attained. As in our discussion earlier in this chapter, pain is not a very good indicator of health. Often times, people are completely unaware of problems that are developing in them because there is no pain associated with them. Consider that heart disease, cancer, and diabetes – the three top killers – don't have any symptoms at all until they have become very advanced. The same is true with cavities in your teeth – there is usually no pain until a cavity becomes severe. The point is that just because you are no longer experiencing pain does not mean that your problem no longer exists. It is important to continue being treated so that the underlying cause of the pain can be corrected.

Routine chiropractic care is one of the simplest ways to maintain the health of your body. Numerous research studies have shown that people who receive regular chiropractic care suffer fewer illnesses, injuries and degenerative diseases, and they report a better overall quality of life. In spite of the health benefits of chiropractic care, many people have never been to a chiropractor, most often because they don't really understand what chiropractic care is all about.

The bottom line is that chiropractic care is a safe, effective treatment for a wide range of physical complaints, such as headaches, neck pain, low back pain, carpal tunnel syndrome, stomach, scoliosis, otitis media, and a host of other problems. While most of these symptoms disappear within a few weeks or months, routine chiropractic care will help ensure full correction of the spine and optimal health for life.

Q. Is chiropractic care safe during pregnancy?

Yes. It is very safe for both mother and baby. Our doctors have advanced training to adjust the pregnant spine. Our adjusting tables have special modifications for pregnant women. Many women utilize the benefits of chiropractic to enjoy health and stress free pregnancies and deliveries.

Q. Is chiropractic safe for babies?

Yes. Improving spinal alignment can benefit people of all ages. It only makes sense that if you have a spine, you should see a spinal expert who is trained to keep your spine healthy. Due to the traumas and stresses of birth, many people bring their newborn babies to get their spines checked for misalignments. Often very gentle adjustments can correct subluxations from birth and help a baby's healthy growth. Doesn't it make sense to correct a problem early in life, rather than suffer from problems after the spine has matured?

2

Low Back Pain and Sciatica

Christy came to my office with terrible lower back pain. She is a petite woman with 4 kids and a newly adopted 80 lb. Labrador retriever. "This problem has been building over time," she complained, "I guess my pushing the stroller and pulling the big dog at the same time has finally taken its toll." Christy is just 36 years old and is feeling her health slipping. She never had lower back pain prior to her pregnancies, saying she used to be fit and active. All the lifting that being a mother of four involves has slowly put pressure on her spine. She feels the pain build all day until the evening when it is unbearable. She describes her lower back problem as extremely achy and stiff, making it very hard to bend. Her goal was obviously to remove the pain, yet a deeper goal was a desire to be an active, fit woman again.

During her exam, I noticed Christy had tightness throughout the muscles of her lower back, especially in the quadratus lumborum muscle, which is located just to the side of the spine in about the middle of the lower back. In addition, her x-rays showed her sacrum (tailbone) was stuck out of place. This kind of subluxation (misalignment) is the most common cause of post-pregnancy lower back pain. We began care at once and Christy noticed an immediate improvement of her condition, although since this problem had been going on since her 8 year old was born, it took some regularity to resolve the issue. Christy is now a regular at the YMCA, her favorite class being the 11 a.m. yoga class. She gets her spine checked periodically, not because she is in pain, but because she never wants to go back to the way it was.

Eighty percent of people suffer from back pain at some point in their lives. Back pain is the second most common reason for visits to the doctor's office, outnumbered only by upper-respiratory infections. In fact, it is estimated that low back pain affects more than half of the adult population each year and more than 10% of all people experience frequent bouts of low back pain. The susceptibility of the low back to injury and pain is due to the fact that the low back, like the neck, is a very unstable part of the spine, unlike the thoracic spine, which is supported and stabilized by the rib cage. This instability allows us to have a great deal of mobility to touch our toes, tie our shoes or pick something up from the ground, but it comes at the cost of increased risk of injury. As long as it is healthy and functioning correctly, the low back can withstand tremendous forces without injury. Professional power lifters can pick up several hundred pounds off the floor without injuring their low back. However, if the low back is out of adjustment or has weakened supporting muscles, something as simple as taking a bag of groceries out of the trunk of the car, picking something up off the floor, or even simply bending down to pet the cat can cause a low back injury.

Until recently, researchers believed that back pain would heal on its own. We have learned, however, that this is not true. Recent studies showed that when back pain is not treated, it may go away temporarily, but will most likely return. It is important to take low back pain seriously and seek professional chiropractic care. This is especially true with pain that recurs over and over again.

The Causes of Low Back Pain

As we talked about earlier, the back is a complicated structure of bones, joints, ligaments, and muscles. You can sprain ligaments, strain muscles, rupture disks, develop trigger points and irritate joints; all of which can lead to back pain. While sports injuries or accidents can lead to injury and pain, sometimes even the simplest movements, like picking up a pencil from the floor, can have painful results. In addition, conditions such as arthritis, poor posture, obesity, psychological stress and even kidney stones, kidney infections, blood clots, or bone loss can also lead to low back pain. Due to the fact that there so many things that can cause low back pain and some of those things can be quite serious if left untreated, it is important to seek professional help. Chiropractors are experts at diagnosing the cause and determining the proper treatment for low back pain. Here are some of the most common causes I see:

Subluxations

As I talked about earlier in this book, whenever there is a disruption in the normal movement or position of the vertebrae, the result is pain and inflammation. In the lumbar spine, these usually occur at the transition between the lower spine and the sacrum. Subluxations can lead to debilitating low back pain. Fortunately, subluxations are easily treatable and often times a significant reduction in pain is experienced almost immediately after the initial treatment.

Disc Herniations

Contrary to popular belief, a herniated disc does not automatically mean that you are going to suffer from low back pain. In fact, one study found that almost half of all adults had at least one bulging or herniated disc, even though they did not suffer any back pain from it. On the other hand, herniated discs can be a source of intense and debilitating pain that frequently radiates to other areas of the body. Unfortunately, once a disc herniates, they rarely, if ever, completely heal. Further deterioration can often be avoided through regular chiropractic care, but a complete recovery is much less common.

Sprains, Strains and Spasms

This is commonly the source of low back pain among the "weekend warriors." You know them. They engage in very little physical activity during the week, but once the weekend arrives, they push themselves way too much. By the end of the weekend, they are lying flat on their back counting down the hours before they can get in to see their chiropractor. Overworking the muscles or ligaments of the low back can lead to small tears in the tissues, which then become painful, swollen and tight.

Sciatica

The sciatic nerve is the longest nerve in your body. It runs from your pelvis, through your hip area and buttocks and down each leg. The sciatic nerve branches into smaller nerves as it travels down the legs, providing feeling to your thighs, legs, and feet as well as controlling many of the muscles in your lower legs. The term sciatica refers to pain that radiates along the path of this nerve. Sciatica is actually a sign that you have an underlying problem putting pressure on a nerve in your lower back. The most common cause of this nerve compression is a bulging or herniated lumbar disc. Piriformis syndrome is another common cause of sciatica. The piriformis is a muscle that lies directly over the sciatic nerve. If this muscle becomes tight or if you have a spasm in this muscle, it puts pressure directly on the sciatic nerve. Other conditions such as lumbar spinal stenosis and spondylolisthesis may also cause nerve compression and nerve irritation resulting in sciatica. Pain that radiates from your lower (lumbar) spine to your buttocks and down the back of your leg is the hallmark of sciatica. Sciatica may be accompanied by numbness, tingling, and muscle weakness in the affected leg. This pain can vary widely, from a mild ache to a sharp, burning sensation or excruciating discomfort. Sometimes it may feel like a jolt or electric shock. Sciatic pain often starts gradually and intensifies over time. It's likely to be worse when you sit, cough or sneeze.

Stress

Whenever you become stressed, your body responds by increasing your blood pressure and heart rate, flooding your body with stress hormones and tightening up your muscles. When you are stressed all the time, the chronic tension causes your muscles to become sore, weak and loaded with trigger points. If you are stressed out all of the time and you have low back pain, it is important to do some relaxation exercises, such as deep breathing, as well as to get regular physical exercise.

Chiropractic Care

Chiropractic treatment for low back pain is usually pretty straightforward. Most commonly, it's simply a matter of adjusting the lower lumbar vertebrae and pelvis to re-establish normal motion and position of your bones and joints. Chiropractic for the low back has been repeatedly shown to be the most effective treatment for low back pain. In fact, major studies have shown that chiropractic care is more effective, affordable and has better long term outcomes than any other treatment.

This makes sense because chiropractic care is the only method of treatment that serves to re-establish normal vertebral motion and position in the spine. All other treatments, such as muscle relaxants, pain killers and bed rest, only serve to decrease the symptoms of the problem and do not correct the problem itself.

In 1999, Blue Cross/Blue Shield (BCBS) of Kansas presented a study of health care statistics of different types of treatment for low back pain. The results showed that chiropractic was more cost-effective than anesthesiology, neurosurgery, neurology, registered physical therapy, orthopedic reconstructive surgery, physical medicine and rehabilitation, and rheumatology. This study confirmed what many others have known in the past – that patients suffering from back problems are much better off going to a chiropractor.

Exercises and Stretches

Back muscles—like any other muscle in the body—require adequate exercise to maintain strength and tone. While muscles in the buttock and thighs are used to walk or climb a flight of stairs, deep back muscles and abdominal muscles are usually left inactive and unconditioned. Unless the back and abdominal muscles are specifically exercised, they will become weak and leave the low back susceptible to injury and pain. Muscle strength and flexibility are essential to maintaining a healthy spine. In the chapter on exercise and stretching, you will find some exercises and stretches that you can do at home to help stabilize and strengthen your low back.

3

Neck and Upper Back Pain

One of my most rewarding cases was a patient that showed up in my clinic complaining of debilitation neck and upper back pain. Bob had been suffering with this problem for 3 years when I met him and he had been through the medical gambit. An MRI had helped in the diagnosing of two disc herniations in his neck. He had been referred to a pain clinic where they injected him with steroid shots for the pain. "It was a horrible treatment," he describes, "after the first injection, I was bedridden, too dizzy to stand and when I did, I passed out!" The shot helped for the short term, yet the severe pain eventually returned. The recommendation was more shots. That is when he came to my clinic. "It feels like someone is driving a nail through my left upper back/shoulder and pain also shoots to my head causing me to have a headache every day," he describes.

His job requires him to drive, work on the computer and travel quite a bit and that only makes things worse. "I am just sick of this! I'm 33 years old and I feel like I am 80." Bob's goals were simple: He wanted the pain to go away and to be able to ride his bike with a back pack again. Bike riding had been out of the question since it brought the pain on immediately.

At his examination, I noticed that he had some posture issues, especially that his head is more forward than it should be on his neck. His muscles in the neck and upper back were in spasm, especially the trapezius and levator scapulae, the muscles that attach your neck to your upper back. The x-rays showed the real cause, an undiagnosed scoliosis in his upper back, probably from childhood. Once he saw this he did admit he has suffered from headaches since childhood.

Once we started adjustments, he immediately noticed relief. He felt the pressure that had been present for years leave his neck and his upper back. His headaches went away as time went on and eventually he even got back to some light exercise. After months of care, I threatened to take him myself to buy a bike. He has sold his car, bought a bike and never felt healthier. His favorite recreation is riding his bike to his volleyball league.

Bob's story is not all that uncommon. Most people do not realize how much they move their neck during the day until they are unable to do so. The degree of flexibility of the neck, coupled with the fact that it has the least amount of muscular stabilization and it has to support and move your 14-16 pound head, means that the neck is very susceptible to injury. You can picture your neck and head much like a bowling ball being held on top of a stick by small, thin, elastic bands. It doesn't take much force to disrupt that delicate balance.

As you read earlier, the spinal cord runs through a space in the vertebrae to send nerve impulses to every part of the body. Between each pair of cervical vertebrae, the spinal cord sends off large bundles of nerves that run down the arms and to some degree, the upper back. This means that if your arm is hurting, it may actually be a problem in the neck! Symptoms in the arms can include numbness, tingling, cold, aching, and "pins and needles." These symptoms can be confused with carpal tunnel syndrome, a painful condition in the hands that is often found in people who work at computer keyboards or perform other repetitive motion tasks for extended periods.

Problems in the neck can also contribute to headaches, muscle spasms in the shoulders and upper back, ringing in the ears, otitis media (inflammation in the middle ear, often mistaken for an ear infection in children), temporo mandibular joint dysfunction (TMJ), restricted range of motion and chronic muscle tightness in the neck and upper back.

We will talk about the neck and upper back together, because most of the muscles that are associated with the neck either attach to, or are located in, the upper back. These muscles include the trapezius, the levator scapulae, the cervical paraspinal muscles, the scalenes, as well as others.

The Causes of Neck and Upper Back Pain

Most neck and upper back pain is caused by a combination of factors, including injury, poor posture, chiropractic subluxations, stress, and in some instances, disc problems.

Injuries

By far, the most common injury to the neck is a whiplash injury. Whiplash is caused by a sudden movement of the head—backward, forward, or sideways—that results in the damage to the supporting muscles, ligaments and other connective tissues in the neck and upper back. Whether from a car accident, sports, or an accident at work, whiplash injuries need to be taken very seriously. Because symptoms of a whiplash injury can take weeks or months to manifest, it is easy to be fooled into thinking that you are not as injured as you really are.

Too often people don't seek treatment following a car accident or sports injury because they don't feel hurt. Unfortunately, by the time more serious complications develop, some of the damage from the injury may have become permanent. Numerous studies have shown that years after whiplash victims settle their insurance claims; roughly half of them state that they still suffer with symptoms from their injuries. If you have been in a motor vehicle or any other kind of accident, please don't assume that you escaped injury if you are not currently in pain. Please get checked out by a chiropractor.

Poor Posture

One of the most common causes of neck pain, and sometimes headaches, is poor posture. It's easy to get into bad posture habits without even realizing it. Even an activity as "innocent" as reading in bed can ultimately lead to pain, headaches, and more serious problems. The basic rule is simple: keep your neck in a "neutral" position whenever possible. Don't bend or hunch your neck forward for long periods. Also, try not to sit in one position for a long time. If you must sit for an extended period, make sure your posture is good: Keep your head in a neutral position, make sure your back is supported, keep your knees slightly lower than your hips, and rest your arms if possible.

Subluxations

Subluxations in the neck and upper back area are extremely common due to the high degree of stress associated with holding up your head, coupled with the high degree of instability in the cervical spine. Most subluxations tend to be centered around four areas: the top of the cervical spine where it meets the skull, in the middle of the cervical spine where the mechanical stress from the head is the greatest, in the transition where the cervical and thoracic areas of the spine meet, and, in the middle of the thoracic spine where the mechanical stress from the weight of the upper body is greatest.

Stress

When most people become stressed, they unconsciously contract their muscles. In particular, they tense muscles in the back and neck. This 'muscle guarding' is a survival response designed to guard against injury. In today's world where we are not exposed to physical danger most of the time, muscle guarding still occurs whenever we become emotionally stressed. The areas most affected are the muscles of the neck, upper back and low back. For most of us, the particular muscle affected by stress is the trapezius muscle, where daily stress usually leads to chronic tightness and the development of trigger points.

The two most effective ways to reduce the physical effects of stress is to increase your activity level – exercise – and deep breathing exercises. By decreasing the physical effects of stress, you can substantially reduce the amount of tightness and pain in your upper back and neck.

Disc Herniations

The discs in your cervical spine can herniate or bulge and put pressure on the nerves that exit from the spine through that area. Although cervical discs do not herniate nearly as often as lumbar discs do, they occasionally can, especially when the discs sustain damage from a whiplash injury.

Treating Neck and Upper Back Pain with Chiropractic

In order to achieve the goal of reducing or eliminating upper back and neck pain, it is necessary to re-establish normal posture, mobility, strength and coordination of the spinal vertebrae, joints and muscles. The most effective way is through chiropractic care. Numerous studies conducted by universities and funded by the U.S. Government have shown repeatedly that chiropractic adjustments are the most effective means of treating problems in the spine, especially in the low back and neck regions. Any treatment of the neck and upper back that neglects chiropractic adjustments of those areas is incomplete.

As described earlier in this chapter, most subluxations tend to be centered around four areas: the top of the cervical spine where it meets the skull; in the middle of the cervical spine where the mechanical stress from the head is the greatest; in the transition where the cervical and thoracic areas of the spine meet; and, in the middle of the thoracic spine where the mechanical stress from the weight of the upper body is greatest.

Each of these subluxated areas are associated with particular symptoms. The upper most subluxations between the cervical spine and the skull tend to cause headaches. The subluxations in the middle of the neck tend to cause neck stiffness and pain. Subluxations at the transition between the cervical and thoracic areas of the spine tends to create chronic muscle tightness and trigger points in the trapezius and levator muscles in the upper back. The subluxations in the middle of the thoracic spine tend to lead to mid back pain, as well as a disruption of normal digestion – indigestion, gastric-esophageal reflux, and gastric ulcers.

Exercises for Your Neck and Upper Back

Because you have to support the weight of your head on top of a highly flexible neck, it is critical that your neck and upper back muscles be flexible and strong. It is important, however, that when you start exercising a particular muscle or muscle group, that it is free from spasms and trigger points in order to avoid irritating the muscle tissue. In Chapter 9, you will learn some very effective exercises and stretches for your neck and upper back. If you have not done these exercises before, be sure to start off slow. Use light pressure initially and build up the intensity over several weeks. This will help you avoid injuries to your muscles, while improving your health.

4

Headaches

Headaches affect just about everyone at some point and they can present themselves in many different ways. Melissa is 23 years old and is someone that has suffered for years with severe migraines. Interestingly this is not the reason for her visit to my clinic. "I always noticed my muscles were tense, even massage therapists would comment on how tight every muscle was in my spine," she confessed at our first meeting. Melissa had woken up with severe back spasms that kept her flat on her back for 5 days. A coworker recommended my clinic.

Upon further discussion, it was revealed that she had been a long sufferer of migraine headaches. She remembers being a cheerleader as a kid and when she was 11 years old, she was dropped on her head during a routine. Her headaches started then. “My headaches always start in my neck and jaw then trigger an intense pain behind my eyes and in my temples,” she explained. She had seen all the specialists and was currently on many medications to try and control the migraines including drugs meant for seizures, beta blockers, and strong painkillers. These drugs slightly controlled the pain yet did not get rid of her headaches. Plus, the side effects made her very shaky and drowsy.

The big thing we noticed when examining her is the amount of tension in her entire spine. She could barely be palpated without jumping in pain and spasm. Her exam showed multiple vertebrae in her neck and upper back were stuck in the wrong position. Her nerves showed severe irritation throughout her whole spine. Melissa was started on adjustments using the ProAdjuster instrument. “I love that thing!” The back spasm she came in with initially went away after a few adjustments.

Her body began to heal and within a few weeks, her headaches began to go away. Once they were a thing of the past, she talked with her medical doctor and they made a plan to wean her off of all the medications. Melissa’s headaches are gone! She is able to be as active and feels her muscles are not nearly as stressed. “My massage therapist couldn’t be happier. She says chiropractic has made her job so much easier,” she exclaimed.

The majority of recurrent headaches are of two types: tension headaches (also called cervicogenic headaches) and migraine headaches. There is a third less common type of headache called a cluster headache, which is a cousin to the migraine. Let's start out by taking a look at each of these three types of headaches.

Tension Headaches

Tension type headaches are the most common, affecting upwards of 75% of all headache sufferers. Most people describe a tension headache as a constant dull, achy feeling either on one or both sides of the head, often described as a feeling of a tight band or dull ache around the head or behind the eyes. These headaches usually begin slowly and gradually and can last for minutes or days, and tend to begin in the middle or toward the end of the day.

Tension headaches are often the result of stress or bad posture, which stresses the spine and muscles in the upper back and neck. Tension headaches, or stress headaches, can last from 30 minutes to several days. In some cases, chronic tension headaches may persist for many months. Although the pain can at times be severe, tension headaches are usually not associated with other symptoms, such as nausea, throbbing or vomiting.

The most common cause of tension headaches is subluxations in the upper back and neck, especially the upper neck, usually in combination with active trigger points. When the top cervical vertebrae lose their normal motion or position, a small muscle called the rectus capitis posterior minor (RCPM) muscle goes into spasm. The problem is that this small muscle has a tendon which slips between the upper neck and the base of the skull and attaches to a thin pain-sensitive tissue called the dura mater that covers the brain. Although the brain itself has no feeling, the dura mater is very pain-sensitive. Consequently, when the RCPM muscle goes into spasm and its tendon tugs at the dura mater, a headache occurs. People who hold desk jobs will tend to suffer from headaches for this reason.

Another cause of tension type headaches comes from referred pain from trigger points in the sternocleidomastoid (SCM) or levator muscle on the side of the neck. These are much more common in people who suffer a whiplash injury due to the muscle damage in the neck region.

Migraine Headaches

Each year, 25 million people in the U.S. experience migraine headaches, 75% being women. Migraines are intense and throbbing headaches that are often associated with nausea and sensitivity to light or noise. They can last from as little as a few hours to as long as a few days. Many of those who suffer from migraines experience visual symptoms called an "aura" just prior to an attack that is often described as seeing flashing lights or that everything takes on a dream-like appearance. Migraine sufferers usually have their first attack before age 30 and they tend to run in families, supporting the notion that there is a genetic component to them. Some people have attacks several times a month, others have less than one a year. Most people find that migraine attacks occur less frequently and become less severe as they get older.

Migraine headaches are caused by a constriction of the blood vessels in the brain, followed by a dilation of blood vessels. During the constriction of the blood vessels there is a decrease in blood flow, which is what leads to the visual symptoms that many people experience. Even in people who don't experience the classic migraine aura, most of them can tell when an attack is imminent. Once the blood vessels dilate, there is a rapid increase in blood pressure inside the head. It is this increased pressure that leads to the pounding headache. Each time the heart beats it sends another shock wave through the carotid arteries in the neck up into the brain.

There are many theories about why the blood vessels constrict in the first place, but no one knows for sure. What we do know is that there are a number of things that can trigger migraines: lack of sleep, stress, flickering lights, strong odors, changing weather patterns and several foods. At the end of this chapter, I have listed a number of foods that are most likely to trigger migraines, as well as some lifestyle changes that you can make to reduce the likelihood that you will trigger a migraine headache.

Cluster Headaches

Cluster headaches are typically very short in duration and excruciating headaches. They are usually felt on one side of the head behind the eyes. Cluster headaches affect about 1 million people in the United States and, unlike migraines, are much more common in men. This is the only type of headache that tends to occur at night. The reason that they are called 'cluster' headaches is that they tend to occur one to four times per day over a period of several days. After one cluster of headaches is over, it may be months or even years, before they occur again. Like migraines, cluster headaches are likely to be related to a dilation of the blood vessels in the brain, causing a localized increase in pressure.

Chiropractic Care for Headaches

Numerous research studies have shown that chiropractic adjustments are very effective for treating tension headaches, especially those that originate in the neck. A report released in 2001 by researchers at the Duke University Evidence-Based Practice Center in Durham, N.C., found that "spinal manipulation resulted in almost immediate improvement for those headaches that originate in the neck, and had significantly fewer side effects and longer-lasting relief of tension-type headaches than commonly prescribed medications." These findings support an earlier study published in the Journal of Manipulative and Physiological Therapeutics that found spinal manipulative therapy to be very effective for treating tension headaches. This study also found that those who stopped chiropractic treatment after four weeks continued to experience a sustained benefit in contrast to those patients who received pain medication.

Each individual's case is different and requires a thorough evaluation before a proper course of chiropractic care can be determined. However, in most cases of tension headaches, significant improvement is accomplished through manipulation of the upper two cervical vertebrae, coupled with adjustments to the junction between the cervical and thoracic spine. This is also helpful in most cases of migraine headaches, as long as food and lifestyle triggers are avoided as well.

Avoid Headache Triggers

- *Stress may be a trigger, but certain foods, odors, menstrual periods, and changes in weather are among many factors that may also trigger headaches.*
- *Emotional factors such as depression, anxiety, frustration, letdown, and even pleasant excitement may be associated with developing a headache.*
- *Keeping a headache diary will help you determine whether factors such as food, change in weather, and/or mood have any relationship to your headache pattern.*
- *Repeated exposure to nitrite compounds can result in a dull, pounding headache that may be accompanied by a flushed face. Nitrite, which dilates blood vessels, is found in such products as heart medicine and dynamite, but is also used as*

a chemical to preserve meat. Hot dogs and other processed meats containing sodium nitrite can cause headaches.

- *Eating foods prepared with monosodium glutamate (MSG) can result in headache. Soy sauce, meat tenderizer, and a variety of packaged foods contain this chemical which is touted as a flavor enhancer.*
- *Headache can also result from exposure to poisons, even common household varieties like insecticides, carbon tetra chloride, and lead. Children who ingest flakes of lead paint may develop headaches. So may anyone who has contact with lead batteries or lead-glazed pottery.*
- *Foods that are high in the amino acid tyramine should also be avoided, such as ripened cheeses (cheddar, brie), chocolate, as well as any pickled or fermented foods.*

5

Pregnancy

Amanda, a pregnant mother of one, had decided that her second pregnancy was going to be different than the first. Her first pregnancy was a caesarean birth due to the baby being breech. Amanda tells us, "Since the birth of my daughter Georgia in 2005, my lower back has not been the same." She continues, "I wanted to be proactive about the back pain and I also wanted to see what I could do to avoid another breech baby. My first baby was breech and while my medical doctor could not find any internal reason for the breech, I was concerned there was a spinal or muscular issue."

Amanda complained of back pain since her first pregnancy and it was increasing with her growing pregnant body. "I feel like my tailbone is out of whack!" That is exactly what the examination found, a sacral subluxation (misalignment). She was also positive for the Webster Technique.

The Webster Technique is a specific chiropractic analysis and adjustment that reduces interference to the nerves and facilitates biomechanical balance in pelvic structures, muscles and ligaments. This has been shown to reduce the effects of intra-uterine constraint, allowing the baby to get into the best possible position for birth. Let Amanda tell you in her own words: "My experience has been really wonderful. I was surprised by the technology that Dr. Maj uses to diagnose muscle and nerve function. I have successfully avoided back pain and have had no swelling or discomfort in my feet. I have been active and have slept well throughout the pregnancy. After the initial scan and two re-examinations, I cannot only feel, but see the results of the chiropractic adjustments. It is really amazing. The final gift was Winifred (Winnie). I am proud to announce that Winnie was a product of a natural birth and was in a perfect birth position. Thanks chiropractic!"

This is an example of why chiropractic care in pregnancy is an essential ingredient to your prenatal care choices. Chiropractic adjustments result in easier pregnancy, significantly decreased the average labor time, and assists new mothers back to prepartum health. In one study, women receiving chiropractic care through their first pregnancy had 24% shorter labor times than the group not receiving chiropractic, and multiparous subjects reported 39% shorter labor times. Thirty-nine percent. That's a massive difference. In addition, 84% of women reported relief of back pain during pregnancy with chiropractic care. Because the sacroiliac joints of the pelvis function better, there is significant less likelihood of back labor when receiving chiropractic care throughout pregnancy.

A large percent of all pregnant women experience back pain during pregnancy. This is due to the rapid growth of the baby and interference to your body's normal structural adaptations to that growth. These pre-existing unnoticed imbalances in your spine and pelvis become overtaxed during pregnancy. The added stresses lead to discomfort and difficulty while performing routine, daily activities. Chiropractic care throughout pregnancy can relieve and even prevent the common discomforts experienced in pregnancy. Specific adjustments eliminate these stresses in your spine, restore balance to your pelvis and result in greater comfort and lifestyle improvements. We will be discussing the importance of the pelvis and spine and its relationship to breech babies later in this chapter and its treatment, The Webster Technique.

As your baby develops, your uterus enlarges to accommodate the rapid growth. So long as the pelvis is in a balanced state, the ligaments connected to the uterus maintain an equalized, supportive suspension for the uterus. If your pelvis is out of balance in any way, these ligaments become torqued and twisted, causing a condition known as constraint to your uterus. This constraint limits the space of the developing baby. Any compromised position for the baby throughout pregnancy will affect his or her optimal development.

Conditions such as torticollis occur because a baby's space was cramped in utero. If the woman's uterus is constrained as birth approaches, the baby is prevented from getting into the best possible position for birth. Even if the baby is in the desirable head down position, often time constraint to the uterus affects the baby's head from moving into the ideal presentation for delivery. The head may be slightly tilted off to one side or even more traumatically, present in the posterior position.

Any baby position even slightly off during birth will slow down labor, and add pain to both the mother and baby. Many women have been told that their babies were too big, or labor "just slowed down" when it was really the baby's presentation interfering with the normal process and progression. Avoidable interventions are implemented turning a natural process into an operative one. Doctors of Chiropractic work specifically with your pelvis throughout pregnancy restoring a state of balance and creating an environment for an easier, safer delivery.

Preparing for a Safer Birth

Dystocia is defined as difficult labor and is something every woman wants to avoid. In addition to the pain and exhaustion caused by long, difficult labors, dystocia leads to multiple medical interventions which may be physically and emotionally traumatic to both you and your baby. Some of these interventions are the administering of pitocin, the use of epidurals, painful episiotomies, forceful pulling on the baby's fragile spine, vacuum extraction, forceps and perhaps even c-sections. Each of these procedures carries a high risk of injury to you, your baby or both! However, all of these procedures used to hasten the delivery process can be avoided if delivery goes more smoothly to begin with. When reviewing the obstetric texts, the reported reasons for dystocia are caused by pelvic imbalance and its resulting effects on your uterus and your baby's position.

Chiropractic care throughout pregnancy restores balance to your pelvic muscles and ligaments and therefore leads to safer and easier deliveries for you and your baby. Additionally, the chiropractic adjustment removes interference to the nervous system allowing your uterus to function at its maximum potential.

The Webster Technique

The Webster Technique benefits all aspects of your body's ability to be healthy. This is accomplished by working with the nervous system—the communication system between your brain and body. Doctors of chiropractic work to correct spinal, pelvic and cranial misalignments (subluxations). When misaligned, these structures create an imbalance in surrounding muscles and ligaments.

Additionally, the resulting nerve system stress may affect the body's ability to function optimally. Sacral misalignment causes the tightening and torsion of specific pelvic muscles and ligaments. It is these tense muscles and ligaments and their constraining effect on the uterus which prevents the baby from comfortably assuming the best possible position for birth.

The Webster Technique is defined as a specific chiropractic analysis and adjustment that reduces interference to the nerve system and facilitates biomechanical balance in pelvic structures, muscles and ligaments. This has been shown to reduce the effects of intrauterine constraint, allowing the baby to get into the best possible position for birth.

Dr. Larry Webster, Founder of the International Chiropractic Pediatric Association, discovered this technique as a safe means to restore proper pelvic balance and function for pregnant mothers. In expectant mothers presenting breech, there has been a high reported success rate of the baby turning to the normal vertex position. This technique has been successfully used in women whose babies present transverse and posterior as well. It has also been successfully used with twins. Any position of the baby other than optimal may indicate the presence of sacral subluxation and therefore intrauterine constraint. At no time should this technique be interpreted as an obstetric "breech turning" technique.

It is strongly recommended by the ICPA instructors of this technique that this specific analysis and adjustment of the sacrum be used throughout pregnancy, to detect imbalance and optimize pelvic biomechanics in preparation for safer, easier births. Because of the effect the chiropractic adjustment has on all body functions by reducing nerve system stress, pregnant mothers should have their spines checked regularly throughout pregnancy, optimizing health benefits for both the mother and baby.

6

Pediatrics

I first met Mia the summer of 2002. Mary, Mia's mom, had just started coming to the clinic to get help for her longstanding neck and back pain due to childhood scoliosis. During one of her first visits, Mary met a patient of mine who was two years old and had her chronic ear infection issue resolved by gentle chiropractic care. What I didn't know about Mary is that she had a three year old daughter, Mia, that had the same issues. Mia had her first ear infection at the age of 6 months. The pediatrician put her on the standard dosage of antibiotics. The ear problem went on and by the age of a year and a half, Mia had been on 6 courses of antibiotics. Standard protocol is to put tubes in a child's ears to drain the fluid and that is what was done with Mia. Her infections went away for about a year. Then her left ear tube fell out and her ear infections returned. She went on a roller coaster of 5 more rounds of antibiotics, was slated to have another tube surgery and maintenance dosages of antibiotics. That is when I met Mary and Mia.

"I didn't know chiropractic could help with Mia's ear infections," Mary began. "We have been following the pediatrician's recommendations and yet we knew there had to be an underlying cause to this problem." She went on to tell me of Mia's birth. "They used her head as a lever to accelerate her birth, pulling and twisting on her little neck." As the consultation continued, she described Mia as a little baby that had her head always turned to one side, was currently very high strung, and rarely slept through the night.

During Mia's exam, I noticed spasm of the muscles in the upper neck and that her head still tended to prefer turning to the left which indicated her first vertebrae was twisted, maybe since birth. We also noted nerve irritation in that upper neck by performing some testing on her nerves with equipment called a Subluxation Station. This technology is wonderful because I need to get a deeper picture of the health of the nerves and spine, yet do not like to x-ray children. All tests led to a diagnosis of vertebral subluxation in the upper cervical spine, the same nerves that open and close the eustacean tube.

We commenced a series of gentle pediatric adjustments. These adjustments use little force (totally different than what is done with adults) due to the fact that the pediatric spine is mostly cartilage, not yet fully calcified into bone. After 3 weeks of regular adjustments, her pediatrician confirmed that both ears were clear. Her ear infections returned once more in those first months of care yet she got sick and got well without antibiotics or any medication. Her body had learned to heal itself. She never got another ear infection.

A question that occurs regularly in my clinic is: "Why should children have chiropractic care?" It is a great question and one that I hope will be answered in great depth in this chapter. More and more parents are seeking chiropractic care for their children. I kind of backed into the whole pediatric practice. I started noticing that when we traced my patient's problems, most would say that the problems started in childhood. So I started seeing teenagers and those kids said their problems started even younger, so I started taking care of toddlers and babies. This chronology lead me to a deeper study of pediatrics and pregnancy.

Why Chiropractic?

My experience has shown that sick adults start out as sick children. Most problems I cared for in my adult patients had a beginning in childhood and even as early as birth. Even so called 'natural' birthing methods can stress an infant's spine and developing nerve system. The resulting irritation to the nerve system caused by spinal and cranial misalignment can be the cause of many newborn health complaints. Colic, breathing problems, nursing difficulties, sleep disturbances, allergic reactions and chronic infections can often be traced to nerve system stress.

Since significant spinal trauma can occur at birth, many parents have their newborns checked right away. As the infant grows, learning to hold up the head, sit, crawl and walk are all activities that affect spinal alignment and are important times to have a child checked by a Doctor of Chiropractic. As the child begins to participate in regular childhood activities like skating or riding a bike, small yet significant spinal misalignments (subluxations) may occur. If neglected, the injuries during this period of rapid growth may lead to more serious problems later in life. Subtle trauma throughout childhood will affect the future development of the spine leading to impaired nervous system function. Any interference to the vital nerve system will adversely affect the body's ability to function at its best.

One of the most common reason parents seek care for their child is trauma from an injury of some sort. These misalignments may or may not result in immediate pain or symptoms. Regular chiropractic checkups can identify potential spinal injury from these traumas, make the correction early in life and help avoid many of the health complaints seen later in adults. Proper spinal hygiene is an important key to better health.

Another sought out reason for care is the resolution of a particular symptom or condition. Parents seek care for conditions such as colic, ear infections, asthma, allergies and headaches (to name a few) because they have heard from other parents that chiropractic care can help.

It is important to understand that the Doctor of Chiropractic does not treat conditions or diseases. The expertise of the chiropractor is in checking the child's spine for misalignments that impair nervous system function therefore affecting overall body function. The bones of the spine, the vertebrae, house and protect the spinal cord. The spinal cord is an extension of the brain and carries information from the brain to the body parts and back to the brain again. Subluxations interfere with the nerves' ability to transmit this vital information.

The nerve system controls and coordinates the function of all the systems in the body: circulatory, respiratory, digestive, hormonal, and immune system. Any aspect of health may be impaired by nerve interference. The chiropractic adjustment restores nerve system function allowing the body the ability to express a greater state of health and well-being.

The doctor of chiropractic will take a case history and perform a chiropractic exam to determine if spinal subluxations exist. Diagnostic tests such as surface EMG or Rolling Thermography are performed to gauge the health of the child's nerves. X-rays are not a regular part of an examination. Chiropractic adjusting procedures are modified to fit a child's size, weight, and unique spinal condition. They are both gentle and specific to the child's developing spinal structures. The amount of force is equal to the amount of force used to test a tomato's freshness or the amount of pressure used with contact lenses on the eye. Most parents report that their children enjoy their chiropractic adjustments and look forward to subsequent visits. They also report that their children experience a greater level of health while under regular chiropractic care.

What Can Chiropractic Do for Your Child?

Why do millions of parents bring their children to Doctors of Chiropractic every year? Is it only for highly dramatic health conditions? Is it only for when my child is hurting? Not at all!!

Chiropractic's purpose is to remove interferences to the natural healing power running through the body. When that power is unleashed the healing that results may be profound.

Today we find more parents bringing their children to chiropractors for day-to-day health concerns we're all familiar with: colds, sore throats, ear infections, fevers, colic, asthma, tonsillitis, allergies, bed-wetting, infections, pains, falls, stomach- aches, and the hundred and one little and big things children go through as they grow up.

Chiropractors Do Not Treat Disease

It's most important to understand that chiropractic is not a treatment for disease. Its purpose is to reduce nerve system stress, a serious and often painless condition most children (and adults) have in their bodies. Nerve system stress interferes with the proper functioning of the nervous system, can weaken internal organs and organ systems, lower resistance, reduce healing potential and set the stage for sickness and disorders of all kinds.

When a chiropractor frees the nervous system from spinal stress, the healing power of the body is unleashed, the immune system works more efficiently, resistance to disease increases, and your child's body functions more efficiently. Your child can then respond to internal and external environmental stresses such as germs, changes in temperature, humidity, toxins, pollen and all the other stresses he/she comes in contact with more efficiently.

So although children with diseases are often brought to the chiropractor, the chiropractor is not treating their diseases but is instead reducing nerve system stress, thus permitting their body's natural healing potential to function at its best.

What Exactly Is Nerve System Stress?

Nerve stress is caused by vertebral subluxations. Subluxations are misalignments or distortions of the spinal column, skull, hips, and related tissues (the structural system) that irritate, stretch, impinge or otherwise interfere with the proper function of the nervous system (brain, spinal cord, spinal nerves and peripheral nerves). Since the nervous system controls all functions of the body, any interference to it can have wide-ranging effects

How Is Nerve System Stress Caused?

Nerve system stress can be caused by physical, chemical and/or emotional stress. Physical stress may start in the womb, with the baby lying in a distorted or twisted manner. Spinal nerve stress in newborns is common today. This may be caused by a traumatic or difficult birth which can introduce great stress to the infant's skull, spinal column and pelvis. Throughout childhood, the normal childhood traumas every child experiences can be a source of spinal and cranial trauma. Most of the time the pain from the initial injury "goes away," however, the damage incurred continues to affect the future function of the child's nerve system.

How Does the Chiropractor Correct Nerve System Stress?

This is accomplished first by analyzing the spinal column and related structures for balance and proper function. Where the spinal column is found to be functioning improperly, the Doctor of Chiropractic performs precise corrective procedures called spinal adjustments.

Using their hands and/or specialized instruments, such as the Pro-Adjuster® to gently and specifically correct those abnormal areas, doctors of chiropractic assist the spine and cranium to regain their intended state of balance and the nerve system is freed from stress. It's all about function!

Today's parents are informed and make their health care choices accordingly. They have become more concerned than ever about the adverse effects drugs have on their children. Parents are hesitant to merely mask symptoms with drugs and are justly worried about their numerous side effects. Parents are increasingly asking, when handed a prescription for a child's recurrent problem, "Is this really all I can do for my child? Isn't there a safer option? How can I restore health?" Today's parents desire to achieve a state of true health—this is leading them to seek health care options which support their children's own natural ability to be healthy.

Chiropractic care is one such option. All children function better with 100% nerve function and deserve the right to express their fullest potential. Chiropractic care for children is safe, gentle and effective. It enhances the body's inborn potential for well-being.

Ear Infections (Otitis Media)

Almost half of all children will suffer from at least one middle ear infection (otitis media) before they're a year old, and two-thirds of them will have had at least one episode by age three. The symptoms of otitis media include ear pain, fever, and irritability.

If you look into the ear of a child who has otitis media, you will be able to see a buildup of fluid behind the ear drum, and the inside of the ear will appear inflamed. Otitis media is caused by either a bacterial or viral infection or frequently results from another illness such as a cold. For many children, it can become a chronic problem, requiring treatment year after year, and putting the child at risk of permanent hearing damage and associated speech and developmental problems.

Otitis media commonly emerges when there is improper drainage of the lymph system in the neck, or when the muscle that is supposed to keep bacteria or viruses from entering the eustacean tubes (the tubes in the back of the throat that lead to the inner ear) doesn't work correctly. While both of these things can happen in adults, it usually does not result in an ear infection for two reasons: First, the shape and the length of the eustacean tubes are different in adults, allowing easier drainage and making it more difficult for bacteria to invade. Second, adults tend to spend more time upright than young children do, which also encourages better drainage and decreases risk of infection.

In either case, the underlying root cause of otitis media is usually a mechanical problem. There is either a reduced or blocked drainage of the neck lymph vessels. Nerve irritation in the neck also causes a spasm in the small muscle that opens and closes the eustacean tube. These problems interfere with the drainage causing the fluid to accumulate. This fluid is where the bacterial growth occurs. Instead of treatment that tries to kill the bacteria or virus, a more natural approach would be to restore normal drainage of the ears and neck lymphatics. This is most effectively done through chiropractic.

Unfortunately, the current treatment of choice for medical doctors is to prescribe oral antibiotics, usually amoxicillin, which can be helpful to get rid of a bacterial infection. But, according to many research studies, antibiotics are often not much more effective than the body's own immune system. And repeated doses of antibiotics can lead to drug-resistant bacteria. Most people have heard about the common practice of placing 'tubes in the ears' to relieve the pressure, and therefore pain, of otitis media. During this surgical procedure, a small opening is made in the eardrum and a small tube is placed in the opening. This opening helps to relieve the pressure in the ear and prevents fluid buildup. After a couple of months, the body pushes the tube out and the hole closes. Although the treatment is often effective, it does not address the underlying cause of the infection, which is the abnormal mechanical functioning of the lymphatics, muscles and nerves.

If your child experiences recurrent ear infections, it is important that you talk to your chiropractor. Doctors of Chiropractic are licensed and trained to diagnose and treat patients of all ages and will use a gentler type of treatment for children. By helping to restore the normal function of the tissues of the neck, there is a reduction in the nerve interference in the upper neck. When the nerve irritation is lowered, it calms the spasm of the muscle that opens and closes the eustacean tube allowing normal drainage of the fluid buildup. Otitis media can usually be significantly reduced or completely eliminated in most children with chiropractic care and without the use of antibiotics and surgery.

Frequently Asked Questions About Children and Chiropractic

Why Chiropractic for Children?

Children are susceptible to trauma in their spines from various activities and events. These micro traumas can subluxate the vertebrae of the spine, placing pressure on their spinal nerves and therefore decreasing their bodies' ability to function normally. Although symptoms, such as pain and malfunction may not show up for years, injury to their nervous system can have a lifetime of damaging effects. The three sports that have been shown to cause the most spinal trauma are gymnastics, wrestling and football.

When Should Children Seek Chiropractic Care?

Children should be checked right after birth because of the potential damaging effects of the birth process. Even the most natural births are somewhat traumatic to the infant and may have "hidden damage." Studies show that many children who experience symptoms of colic, ear infections and asthma have spinal subluxations impairing their nervous system function. Early detection and correction can prevent layers of damage from occurring in the child's vital nervous system. Accumulated damage will have lifelong consequences.

Do Chiropractic Adjustments Hurt?

Chiropractors specializing in children use very specific, gentle techniques to care for children. On the very young, the adjustment is as light as a finger touch. Doctors of Chiropractic who are members of the International Chiropractic Pediatric Association have taken post-graduate classes on specific techniques for pregnant mothers, infants and children to enhance their skills in this field.

Most of the members of the International Chiropractic Pediatric Association offer complimentary consultations, giving parents the opportunity to meet them, find out about chiropractic for their families and discuss their individual needs. Visit their website: www.icpa4kids.org.

How Safe is Chiropractic for Children?

A survey study examining the pediatric care of chiropractors in the Boston area estimated that approximately 420,000 pediatric chiropractic visits were made in the Boston metropolitan area alone for 1998. If extrapolated for the rest of the United States and Canada, the number of chiropractic visits to children in one year would be enormous, numbering in several million visits. Given this high utilization rate of pediatric chiropractic services in the United States and Canada, statistics show little evidence of harm to children from chiropractic care.

When the Canadian Pediatric Society published their position statement on, "Chiropractic Care for Children: Controversies and Issues," they addressed the issue of "The Safety of Chiropractic in Pediatrics," they further readily admit that, "Reports of other pediatric complications are few." To put this in perspective: It's been estimated that the annual cost of medication-related problems in the United States is approximately $84.6 billion. The human impact of non-steroidal anti-inflammatory-related gastrointestinal deaths have been estimated at rates higher than that found from deaths due to cervical cancer, asthma or malignant melanoma.

Medication errors and adverse drug events are three times higher in children and substantially higher still for babies. There is a growing use of stimulants, antidepressants and antipsychotic drugs in children as young as 2-4 years of age. The list could go on. Chiropractic for children is here to stay. Millions of children and their families will continue to experience the benefits of this safe and effective form of healthcare called chiropractic. Chiropractic researchers are looking into the positive effects of chiropractic care in children with subluxations and related conditions like ADHD, asthma, colic and others.

Chiropractic Safety and Effectiveness Studies for Children

Lee AC, Li DH, Kemper KJ. Chiropractic care for children. Arch Pediatr Adolesc Med 2000;154:401-407. Canadian Chiropractic Association - www.cps.ca/english/index.htm

Hondras MA, Linde K, Jones AP. Manual therapy for asthma (Cochrane Review). Cochrane Database Syst Rev 2001;1: CD001002.

Johnson JA, Bootman JL. Drug-related morbidity and mortality. A cost-of-illness model. Arch Intern Med 1995;155:1949-1956.

Bates DW, Spell N, Cullen DJ, Burdick E, Laird N, Petersen LA, Small SD, Sweitzer BJ, Leape LL. The costs of adverse drug events in hospitalized patients. Adverse Drug Events Prevention Study Group. JAMA 1997;277:307-311.

Singh G.Gastrointestinal complications of prescription and over-the-counter nonsteroidal anti-inflammatory drugs: a view from the ARAMIS database. Arthritis, Rheumatism, and Aging Medical Information System.Am J Ther. 2000;7:115-121.

Kaushal R, Bates DW, Landrigan C, McKenna KJ, Clapp MD, Federico F, Goldmann DA. Medication errors and adverse drug events in pediatric inpatients. JAMA 2001;285:2114-2120.

Zito JM, Safer DJ, DosReis S, Gardner JF, Boles M, Lynch F. Trends in the prescribing of psychotropic medications to preschoolers. JAMA 2000;23:1025-1030.

7

Vital Step Two: Achieve an Ideal Weight with a Healthy Diet

In my undergraduate work at Ohio University, I studied Clinical Nutrition. I have always had a strong belief that our nutrition plays a MAJOR role in the journey to wellness. The reason I did not go further in this field is that there is always a fad diet out there or some celebrity telling you this is the only way to eat to lose weight. All the books out there are not about getting well, they are about losing weight at whatever cost to the body. Little did I know that in my clinic we would talk as much about nutrition as we do about Chiropractic. It is important to remember that you are what you eat, literally. The food you eat is broken down to make YOU!

I encourage you to choose to eat in a way that can be done for a lifetime. If you are trying to lose weight by an all soup, protein, or broccoli plan, you might lose weight in the short term but your health will suffer and you will most likely gain that weight back in the long term.

Epidemic of Obesity

If you are overweight, you are certainly not alone. Obesity in the United States has become the greatest health crisis of our time; it affects more Americans than any other condition. In 2012, The World Health Statistics came out with new research stating that one in six adults are obese, one in three are hypertensive, and one in 10 are diabetic.

Since 1980, obesity rates have doubled among children and tripled among adolescents. The World Health Organization projects that by 2025, 45% - 50% of all U.S. adults and 30% of all U.S. children will suffer from obesity.

There are many theories as to why this is occurring, including a sedentary lifestyle, consuming too much food, toxins in the environment, genetics, stress, depression, or food additives such as MSG. Most likely it is a combination of all these, so overcoming the problem of obesity will require a comprehensive approach of dietary changes, increased activity levels and nutritional supplementation.

Being Overweight Affects Everything

Being overweight not only affects how you look and feel, it is also detrimental to your overall health. Obesity is a major contributor to many chronic diseases and conditions, including Type II diabetes, hypertension, heart disease, stroke, breast cancer, colon cancer, gallbladder disease, depression and arthritis. And being overweight not only affects you, it also places a huge strain on the total health care system.

In 2003, the total cost of obesity in the United States was estimated at $137 billion, of which $75 billion was for direct medical costs and $62 billion was for indirect costs. That expense boils down to a cost of approximately $350 per year for every single American adult. In fact, the cost in death, disability and lost productivity from obesity has come close to that of tobacco. Those who are obese suffer 30% - 50% more health problems than smokers or problem drinkers.

Metabolic Syndrome

In an article appearing in the January 16, 2002, issue of the Journal of the American Medical Association, researchers at the Centers for Disease Control and Prevention (CDC) estimated that as many as 47 million Americans may exhibit a cluster of medical conditions (a "metabolic syndrome") characterized by insulin resistance, the presence of obesity, abdominal fat, high blood sugar, elevated triglycerides, high blood cholesterol, and high blood pressure.

The root causes of metabolic syndrome for a majority of individuals may be poor diet and insufficient physical activity. Currently, the most effective way to avoid or overcome metabolic syndrome is through a comprehensive program of diet and exercise. Below we are going to discuss in detail how to rewire your metabolism for achieving weight-loss and ultimately an ideal weight for a lifetime.

Creating a New Energy Management System for Ideal Weight

First we need to understand that not all carbohydrates have the same effect on blood glucose (also known as blood sugar) levels. Starches (like in whole grains) are much larger molecules than sugars and therefore take longer to break down and enter the blood stream as glucose. Sugars, on the other hand, are simple molecules that can quickly be converted into glucose and enter the blood. Sugar will tend to create a sharp spike in blood glucose levels, whereas starches will tend to cause a much more gradual increase.

A high glycemic index (GI) carbohydrate is one that causes a very rapid and substantial increase in blood sugar. Foods such as ice cream, cake, sugared breakfast cereals and candy bars fall into the category of high glycemic index foods. Surprisingly, so do many foods that are commonly considered healthy, such as bananas, orange juice, pineapple and watermelon.

Low glycemic index foods are those that have a much lower and slower effect on your body's blood glucose levels. This includes high protein foods, such as meat and eggs, as well as beans, legumes, most vegetables and high-fiber whole grain

The Glycemic Index of Common Foods

Low Glycemic Index Foods (55 or less)

- most vegetables
- yogurt
- oats
- apples

Medium Glycemic Index Foods (56-69)

- potato chips
- Wheat Thins®
- oats
- pineapple

High Glycemic Index Foods (70 or more)

- breakfast cereals
- white bread
- baked potato
- bagel

foods. When your diet consists of a lot of high glycemic index foods, your body will secrete an excess amount of insulin in an effort to keep your blood sugar levels down. This causes much of the carbohydrate you consume to be stored directly into your fat cells, leading to an increase in body fat.

The Main Obstacle to Weight Loss: Insulin Resistance

The other serious detrimental effect of these spikes in blood sugar and spikes in insulin has to do with the fact that when your insulin levels peak at high levels several times per

Glycemic Index and Type II Diabetes

A high glycemic index (GI) carbohydrate is one that causes a very rapid and substantial increase in blood sugar. Foods such as ice cream, cake, sugared breakfast cereals and candy bars fall into the category of high glycemic index foods. Surprisingly, so do many foods that are commonly considered healthy, such as bananas, orange juice, pineapple and watermelon.

Low glycemic index foods are those that have a much lower and slower effect on your body's blood glucose levels. This includes high protein foods, such as meat and eggs, as well as beans, legumes, most vegetables and high-fiber whole grain foods. When your diet consists of a lot of high glycemic index foods, your body will secrete an excess amount of insulin in an effort to keep your blood sugar levels down. This causes much of the carbohydrate you consume to be stored directly into your fat cells, leading to an increase in body fat.

The other serious detrimental effect of these spikes in blood sugar and spikes in insulin has to do with the fact that when your insulin levels peak at high levels several times per day, your muscles and liver, which are important for storing blood glucose, stop reacting to the insulin's message to store some of the sugar that is floating around in the blood. This phenomenon is called insulin resistance.

When insulin resistance develops, your body produces insulin in response to your blood sugar rising, but your body no longer uses the insulin properly, causing your blood sugar levels to remain high. Insulin resistance not only contributes to being overweight, but it is also is the precursor for a serious condition called Type II, or adultonset, diabetes.

The four most effective ways to combat insulin resistance are to consume only low glycemic index foods, eat smaller meals more frequently throughout the day, supplement with chromium and alphalipoic acid, and perform some aerobic exercise each day.

day, your muscles and liver, which are important for storing blood glucose, stop reacting to the insulin's message to store some of the sugar that is floating around in the blood. This phenomenon is called insulin resistance.

When insulin resistance develops, your body produces insulin in response to your blood sugar rising, but your body no longer uses the insulin properly, causing your blood sugar levels to remain high. Insulin resistance not only contributes to being overweight, but it is also the precursor for a serious condition called Type II, or adult-onset, diabetes.

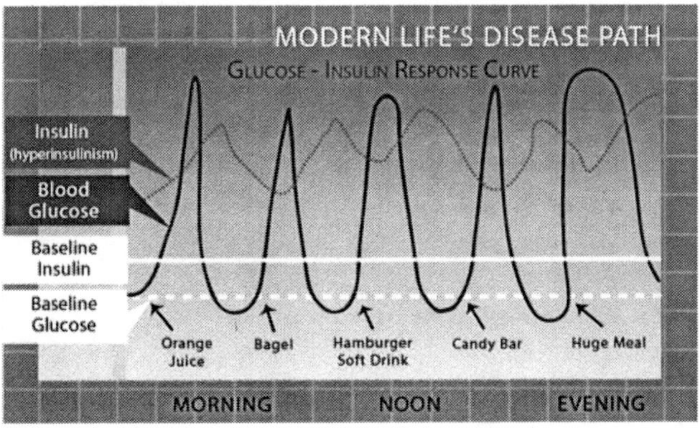

As you can see above, the typical Western diet of highly processed, high glycemic foods – soft drinks, candy bars (or sports bars which are pretty much the same), bagels - cause blood sugar (also known as blood glucose) to rise dramatically. And that makes the level of insulin rise. What happens next is interesting – the elevated insulin level actually causes blood sugar to plummet, creating the rapid rise and fall you see in the chart.

As blood sugar falls below normal, the brain sets off a series of messages that cause cravings – so you start scrambling for something sweet and full of calories. And so the cycle of high and low blood sugar continues, reinforcing eating patterns that lead to poor health and obesity.

When insulin levels stay elevated in this way, the body continues using glucose as fuel, rather than both glucose and fat. And when it is not used as energy, all that ingested fat – along with excess glucose and high fructose corn syrup – is laid down in fat cells. In short, you become a fat storage factory! On top of which, that huge meal right before bed keeps your body in fat-storage mode through the night and disrupts your sleep, leading to even poorer eating habits and more weight gain.

Blood Glucose, Insulin and Glucagon

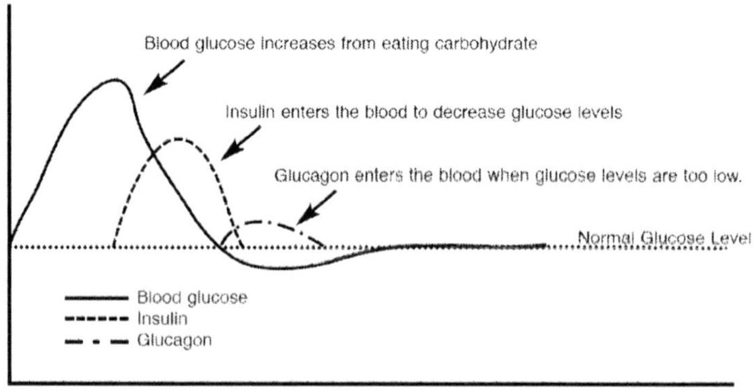

The Myth of Three Squares

A study by David Jenkins, MD, PhD, a University of Toronto pioneer in low-glycemic eating, demonstrates that eating small portions at frequent intervals is good for your health in a number of important, even remarkable, ways.

The researchers divided their subjects into two groups. Both ate the exact same foods with the exact same number of calories. But one group had their food divided into the usual three meals a day. The other ate more often, consuming lots of little meals.

Surprisingly, the group that ate small meals throughout the day lost more weight. They lost weight because their blood sugar didn't continually spike and then dip down to an even level, the way it does after a big meal. Their glycemic levels – the amount of sugar in their blood – remained steady and their cravings for sweet foods went down.

That is not all. After only two weeks, they found that the people who ate every three hours reduced their blood cholesterol by over 15% and their blood insulin by almost 28%. That's the key – because in addition to regulating your blood sugar level, insulin plays a role in fat metabolism, inflammation, and the progression of metabolic syndrome.

So what does this study tell us? That it's not what you eat; it's when you eat it. Small amounts of nourishment throughout the day are better than the same amount of food concentrated in three big hits. Your body begins to work differently, and you are no longer the fat factory you once were.

So now we know that eating smaller, low-glycemic meals is a great way to turn off insulin and provide healthier fuel for our body. What else can help us achieve life-long weight loss?

The Keys to Healthy Weight Loss

What's the key to the successful mastery of both weight loss and long-term health? There are really two main components:

1. The ability to master the amount of fuel you take in.
2. The quality of that fuel.

So if we can devise a plan that delivers lower-calorie, nutrient dense foods in the proper proportions, we have a recipe for success. Low glycemic foods are those that have a much lower and slower effect on your body's blood glucose levels. This includes high protein foods, such as meat and eggs, as well as beans, legumes, most vegetables and high-fiber whole grain foods.

How does it work? Portion size is key. When you eat healthy foods - that is, low-glycemic carbohydrate, healthy fats, and high-quality proteins – in smaller portions than your body is used to, a magical transformation occurs. Your body turns to Plan B and begins to utilize the unhealthy fat around your middle to make up the deficit. The storage system of fat begins to be used as it was intended, providing your body with a constant source of calories while signaling it to turn off insulin, hunger, and cravings for carbohydrates.

And there's another great benefit. By providing your body with these nutrient-dense, protein-rich feedings in small portions throughout the day, you protect your muscles from being cannibalized, unlike in some low-calorie weight-loss programs. But that doesn't mean you won't see results. In fact, you can expect to lose between two and five pounds each week – and after about the first week, it is going to be mostly fat. (During the first week or so of weight loss, you lose excess water weight as well as fat. The good news is that your puffiness will disappear!)

But this efficient, safe platform not only carries you through your initial weight-loss phase, it also sets the stage for a whole new pattern of healthy eating – for LIFE! Let's see how your body is going to respond to this new healthy fueling strategy.

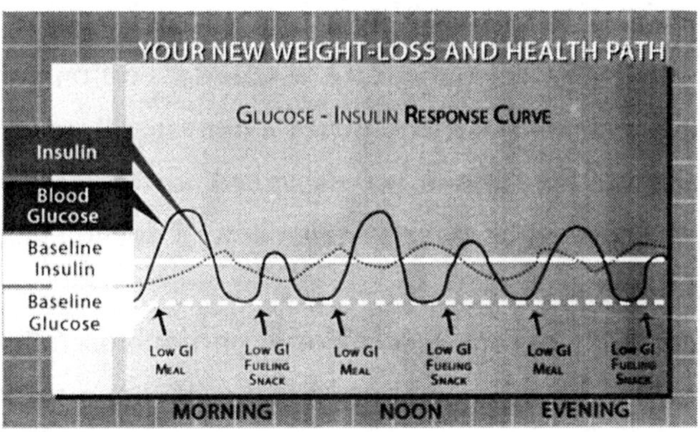

That's a whole different picture than before (see Modern Life's Disease Path earlier in this chapter). First, we've reduced your total energy intake by introducing smaller, portion controlled meals and snacks. Second, we've switched to low-glycemic meals that keep your blood sugar and insulin levels from spiking. This constant stable energy source means no more wide swings in blood sugar. You've turned off your insulin pump and taken control of cravings!

Eating this way – six fuelings, every three hours, starting with a healthy breakfast – helps you build a whole new energy management system, one that disperses energy throughout the day in accord with your body's natural design. Six fuelings helps to offload excess calories, producing the perfect internal environment for hunger control and weight loss.

Catalyst to Reaching a Healthy Weight: Medically Formulated Portion-Controlled Meal Replacements

For quick, effective weight loss without a lot of preparation, medically formulated, low-calorie portion-controlled meal replacements (PCMRs) offers a convenient, ready to use food system in the form of pre-packaged, low glycemic meals. In fact, the success of these systems is well documented in the medical literature.

Medically proven low calorie portion-controlled meal replacements have undergone significant improvements in the last few decades. I believe these meals are on the verge of becoming an integral part of many of our lives. Why? PCMRs are a powerful tool – not as a complete diet in and of themselves, but as a part of a comprehensive approach to healthy eating. PCMRs are the new healthy fast food for the 21st Century!

The PCMR that I use successfully, and that I've helped others experience with success, is made by Medifast®. Medifast's meal replacements set the gold standard, with nearly thirty years of efficacy and safety, backed by studies conducted by researchers from prestigious institutions such as Johns Hopkins University School of Medicine and recommended by over 15,000 physicians since 1980.

Medifast as the preferred PCMRs have many benefits:

- *They are cost effective, because you will be replacing your groceries and snacks with PCMRs, you'll be spending the same or even less than you are now on food.*
- *They offer plenty of variety. Medifast helps you fight fatigue with lots of great-tasting options. There are over 80 foods to choose from.*
- *They help control your calories. New developments in these PCMRs allows for an advanced nutritional footprint to keep you in a fat-burning state while protecting muscle.*

Healthy fast food for the 21st Century. Although patients are initially apprehensive about using meal replacements, the one thing they enjoy the most are these Medifast meals. I always challenge them to prepare 5 meals all containing low glycemic foods with the right proportion of nutrients and measuring around 100 calories per serving. Good luck with that!

Be Slim for Life

Achieving your ideal weight is the first milestone on a path to creating optimal health for a lifetime. How do we maintain this ideal weight? Best to ask people who have been successful in doing just that.

The National Weight Control Registry (NWCR), established in 1994 by Rena Wing, Ph.D. from Brown Medical School, and James O. Hill, Ph.D. from the University of Colorado, is the largest prospective investigation of long-term successful weight loss maintenance. Given the prevailing belief that few individuals succeed at long-term weight loss, the NWCR was developed to identify and investigate the characteristics of individuals who have succeeded at long-term weight loss. The NWCR is tracking over 10,000 individuals who have lost significant amounts of weight and kept it off for long periods of time. They have found six elements that are critical for lifetime success:

- *Eating Breakfast*
- *Regular Exercise*
- *Support*
- *Low fat meals every three hours*
- *Individual plan*
- *Monitoring weight*

Now that you've solidified your understanding of these key habits of health, I truly believe that following these basic rules will begin the process of weight loss while learning to eat healthy for a lifetime. Remember, weight loss is the beginning of a lifelong goal of healthy eating.

For more information regarding these specialized programs, go to youcanbewell.tsfl.com. I can help you finally achieve this vital step to wellness!

8

Vital Step Three: Beat Stress

Modern life is full of pressure, stress and frustration. I live in Chicago and the pace of life there wears many people down. Worrying about your job security, being overworked, driving in rush-hour traffic, arguing with your spouse or partner—all these create stress. According to a recent survey by the American Psychology Association, over half of all Americans are concerned about the level of stress in their everyday lives and two-thirds of Americans say they are likely to seek help for stress. Most people are feeling overscheduled, over extended, and overstressed. By far, the most commonly reported source of stress in people's lives is workplace stress.

A Northwestern National Life study found that one in four employees rank their jobs as the greatest source of stress in their lives. And according to Gallup, 80% of employees suffer from job stress and nearly 40% reporting that they need help in managing their stress. According to the Princeton Survey Research study, three-quarters of employees believe that there is more on-the-job stress than a generation ago.

You may feel physical stress as the result of too much to do, not enough sleep, a poor diet or the effects of an illness. Stress can also be mental: when you worry about money, a loved one's illness, retirement, or experience an emotionally devastating event, such as the death of a spouse or partner or being fired from work.

However, much of our stress comes from less dramatic everyday responsibilities. Obligations and pressures which are both physical and mental are not always obvious to us. In response to these daily strains your body automatically increases blood pressure, heart rate, respiration, metabolism, and blood flow to your muscles. This response is intended to help your body react quickly and effectively to a high-pressure situation. Let's learn about stress, its effects on the body and strategies to reduce it.

The Stress Response

Often referred to as the "fight-or-flight" reaction, the stress response occurs automatically when you feel threatened. Your body's fight-or-flight reaction has strong biological roots. It's there for self-preservation. This reaction gave early humans the energy to fight aggressors or run from predators and was important to help the human species survive. But today, instead of protecting you, it may have the opposite effect. If you are constantly stressed you may actually be more vulnerable to life-threatening health problems.

Any sort of change in life can make you feel stressed, even good change. It's not just the change or event itself, but also how you react to it that matters. What may be stressful is different for each person. For example, one person may not feel stressed by retiring from work, while another may feel stressed.

How stress affects your body

When you experience stress, your pituitary gland responds by increasing the release of a hormone called adrenocorticotropic hormone (ACTH). When the pituitary sends out this burst of ACTH, it's like an alarm system going off deep inside your brain. This alarm tells your adrenal glands, situated atop your kidneys, to release a flood of stress hormones into your bloodstream, including cortisol and adrenaline. These stress hormones cause a whole series of physiological changes in your body, such as increasing your heart rate and blood pressure, shutting down your digestive system and altering your immune system. Once the perceived threat is gone, the levels of cortisol and adrenaline in your bloodstream decline, and your heart rate and blood pressure and all of your other body functions return to normal.

If stressful situations pile up one after another, your body has no chance to recover. This long-term activation of the stress-response system can disrupt almost all your body's processes. Some of the most common physical responses to chronic stress are:

- *Digestive system. Stomach aches or diarrhea are very common when you're stressed. This happens because stress hormones slow the release of stomach acid and the emptying of the stomach. The same hormones also stimulate the colon, which speeds the passage of its contents.*
- *Immune system. Chronic stress tends to dampen your immune system, making you more susceptible to colds and other infections. Typically, your immune system responds to infection by releasing several substances that cause inflammation. Chronic systemic inflammation contributes to the development of many degenerative diseases.*
- *Nervous system. Stress has been linked with depression, anxiety, panic attacks and dementia. Over time, the chronic release of cortisol can cause damage to several structures in the brain. Excessive amounts of cortisol can also cause sleep disturbances and a loss of sex drive.*
- *Cardiovascular system. As mentioned earlier, stress causes an increase in both heart rate and blood pressure and increases the risk of heart attacks and strokes.*

Exactly how you react to a specific stressor may be completely different from anyone else. Some people are naturally laid-back about almost everything, while others react strongly at the slightest hint of stress. If you have had any of the following conditions, it may be a sign that you are suffering from stress:

- *Anxiety*
- *Back pain*
- *Constipation or diarrhea*
- *Depression*
- *Fatigue*
- *Weight gain or loss*
- *Insomnia*
- *Relationship problems*
- *Shortness of breath*
- *Stiff neck*
- *Upset stomach*

Lifestyle Solutions

After decades of research, it is clear that the negative effects associated with stress are real. Although you may not always be able to avoid stressful situations, there are a number of things that you can do to reduce the effect that stress has on your body. The first is relaxation. Learning to relax doesn't have to be difficult. Here are some simple techniques to help get you started on your way to tranquility.

Alignment

One of the consequences of stress is a tendency to unconsciously tense up our muscles – especially in the upper back and abdominal region. This chronic tension, often coupled with poor posture, frequently causes the vertebrae of the spine to become misaligned. As you have read in previous chapters, we call that a subluxation. This subluxation (misalignment) causes irritation of the spinal nerves, and this irritation, in turn, often leads to more muscle tension. In this way, muscle tension becomes both the cause and the consequence of stress – all the while, the misalignments of the spine worsen. This vicious circle will continue until the affected area of the spine is realigned. Unfortunately, there is no way to do this on your own and requires the care of a spinal alignment specialist – the Chiropractor. Most people experience a noticeable improvement in their stress almost immediately after a spinal adjustment.

Healthy Thinking

Just as negative emotions can weaken the body's resistance, positive emotions can strengthen it, or at least allow it to function normally. The simple fact of deciding to be happier and focus on the positive will improve your health. In fact, this phenomenon of your thoughts affecting your physical health is so strong that all medical studies have to be designed with it in mind. Research calls this phenomenon the 'placebo effect.'

Many people believe that the term 'placebo effect' means that the effect is only imagined – that it is not real. But this couldn't be further from the truth. Medical studies have to include a control group – people who receive placebos instead of the medicine being studied – because the simple act of people making the decision to take to improve their health leads to measurable physical improvement in their condition.

To determine how much of the effect a particular medicine had, the researchers have to take the measured change in the group who underwent the particular therapy and subtract out the amount of change seen in the placebo group. Otherwise, there is no way to know whether a particular treatment was beneficial or whether it was merely the change in attitude in the study subjects that made the difference. In many instances, the placebo effect turns out to be stronger than the treatment itself!

The point is that if you want to have a healthy body you also have to have healthy thoughts and emotions. Just as it is important to avoid toxic chemicals, it is also necessary to avoid toxic thoughts to enjoy optimal health.

Relaxed Breathing

Have you ever noticed how you breathe when you're stressed? Stress typically causes rapid, shallow breathing. This kind of breathing sustains other aspects of the stress response, such as rapid heart rate and perspiration. If you can get control of your breathing, the spiraling effects of acute stress will automatically become less intense. Relaxed breathing, also called diaphragmatic breathing, can help you.

Practice this basic technique twice a day, every day, and whenever you feel tense. Follow these steps:

- *Inhale. With your mouth closed and your shoulders relaxed, inhale as slowly and deeply as you can to the count of six. As you do that, push your stomach out. Allow the air to fill your diaphragm.*
- *Hold. Keep the air in your lungs as you slowly count to four.*
- *Exhale. Release the air through your mouth as you slowly count to six.*
- *Repeat. Complete the inhale-hold-exhale cycle three to five times, twice per day.*

Progressive Muscle Relaxation

The goal of progressive muscle relaxation is to reduce the tension in your muscles. First, find a quiet place where you'll be free from interruption. Loosen tight clothing and remove your glasses or contacts if you'd like. Tense each muscle group for at least five seconds and then relax for at least 30 seconds. Repeat before moving to the next muscle group. The following is an example of a progressive relaxation session:

- *Face. Lift your eyebrows toward the ceiling, feeling the tension in your forehead and scalp, then squint your eyes and squish your face in as tight as you can. Relax. Repeat.*

- *Neck. Gently touch your chin to your chest. Feel the pull in the back of your neck as it spreads into your head. Relax. Repeat.*
- *Shoulders. Pull your shoulders up toward your ears, feeling the tension in your shoulders, head, neck and upper back. Relax. Repeat.*
- *Arms. Pull your arms back and press your elbows in toward the sides of your body. Try not to tense your lower arms. Feel the tension in your arms, shoulders and into your back. Relax. Repeat.*
- *Chest, shoulders and upper back. Pull your shoulders back as if you're trying to make your shoulder blades touch. Relax. Repeat.*
- *Stomach. Pull your stomach in toward your spine, tightening your abdominal muscles. Relax. Repeat.*
- *Legs. Squeeze your knees together and lift your legs up off the chair or from wherever you're relaxing. Feel the tension in your thighs. Relax. Repeat.*
- *Feet. Turn your feet inward and curl your toes up and out. Relax. Repeat.*

Each progressive relaxation session should last about 10 minutes and should be performed at least once a day for maximum benefit.

Listen to Soothing Sounds

If you have about 10 minutes and a quiet room, you can take a mental vacation almost anytime. Consider these two types of relaxation CDs or tapes to help you unwind, rest your mind or take a visual journey to a peaceful place.

- *Spoken word. These CDs use spoken suggestions to guide your meditation, educate you on stress reduction or take you on an imaginary visual journey to a peaceful place.*
- *Soothing music or nature sounds. Music has the power to affect your thoughts and feelings. Soft, soothing music can help you relax and lower your stress level.*

No one CD works for everyone, so try several CDs to find which works best for you. When possible, listen to samples in the store. Consider asking your friends or a trusted professional for recommendations.

Exercise

Exercise is a good way to deal with stress because it is a healthy way to relieve your pent-up energy and tension. It also helps you get in better shape, which makes you feel better overall. By getting physically active, you can decrease your levels of anxiety and stress and elevate your moods. Numerous studies have shown that people who begin exercise programs demonstrate a marked improvement in their ability to concentrate, sleep better, have fewer illnesses, experience less pain and report a much higher quality of life than those who do not exercise. This is even true of people who had not begun an exercise program until they were in their 40s, 50s, 60s or even 70s. So if you want to feel better and improve your quality of life, get active!

9

Vital Step Four: Exercise as a Nutrient

Many health experts state that the role of exercise in any weight loss program is simply to burn calories. Their reasoning is that if you burn more calories than you eat, you will lose weight. But, if you don't burn as many calories as you eat, you will gain weight. Simple enough, right?

Although this reasoning makes sense and is true for the most part, it fails to capture the expanse of physiological and mental changes that occur when you exercise. Losing weight is just the tip of the iceberg. I think of exercise as a nutrient, just like vitamin C. Without it your body cannot be well. Exercise also improves your blood pressure, decreases your cholesterol level, decreases your risk of heart disease and cancer, improves your mental functioning, elevates your mood, improves your quality of sleep, keeps you from losing muscle during weight loss, decreases your emotional and physical response to stress and improves your flexibility and balance. In this chapter you will learn how exercise can improve so many aspects of your life, as well as simple ways to integrate exercise into your busy schedule.

Exercise -The Fountain of Youth

In their landmark book entitled Biomarkers, medical researchers Dr. William Evans and Dr. Irwin Rosenberg identified ten characteristic changes that occur as we age, including: a loss of muscle mass, a decrease in strength, a decrease in basal metabolic rate, a decrease in aerobic capacity, an increase in blood pressure, a loss of normal insulin action, a decrease in circulating HDL to total cholesterol ratio, a loss of bone density and a decreased ability to control your body temperature. Each one of these measures of physical health tends to decline as we age. What Evans and Rosenberg discovered is that exercise was effective in reversing every single one of these markers of aging!

To those of the baby boomer generation, the name Jack LaLanne is synonymous with fitness. He hosted his own exercise television show for 34 years beginning in the early 1960s. Jack LaLanne was a sugar-addicted weakling for most of his youth, and at one point, the family doctor had told his parents that he may not have very long to live due to his ill health. One day that changed when Jack decided that he was going to quit eating junk food and begin exercising.

Over the ensuing years, Jack accomplished what many would consider impossible feats, such as performing 1,033 push-ups in 23 minutes on national TV at the age of 42, and on his 70th birthday, swimming 1.5 miles in San Francisco Bay while pulling 70 boats! At 93 years of age, he still exercises for two hours every day - one hour of swimming and one hour of weightlifting.

You don't have to train as intensely as Jack LaLanne in order to enjoy the benefits of exercise. But you do have to get up and get your body moving at least five or six days per week; preferably doing a combination of aerobic exercise and strength training.

The Benefits of Aerobic Exercise

Aerobic means "using oxygen" and aerobic exercises are those that utilize oxygen during the activity. Aerobic exercise trains the body to utilize oxygen more efficiently and improves your overall cardiovascular fitness. Aerobic activities are those that are performed for an extended period of time at a low intensity. Examples of aerobic activities are biking, aerobic walking, swimming, jogging, in- line skating, aerobic dance, cross-country skiing and using an elliptical trainer. The benefits of aerobic activity include:

- *Improved breathing*
- *Increased energy throughout the day*
- *Improved heart health and cardiac output*
- *Decreased blood pressure*
- *Decreased serum cholesterol*
- *Decreased stress*
- *More restful sleep*
- *Improved mood and mental functioning*
- *Improved digestion and bowel function*

For maximum benefit, you should engage in at least 20 minutes of aerobic activity five or six days per week. If you can already do more than this, great! For those who have not engaged in regular activity for a while, even 20 minutes a day will be an accomplishment.

During aerobic exercise, you should be able to carry on a conversation without feeling too winded. If you are breathing too heavy to carry on a conversation easily, you should ease up a bit. As you become healthier, you will be able to increase the intensity of your activity without feeling short of breath.

This brings up another important point - a concept called the overload principle. The overload principle simply states that in order to benefit from physical activity, the intensity has to be greater than your body is used to. Only by pushing your body a little bit - by overloading it - will your body respond by growing stronger.

Staying in the Aerobic Training Zone

The easiest way to tell if you are exercising intensely enough is to measure your heart rate. Your target aerobic heart rate range is calculated by subtracting your age from 220 to find your maximum heart rate for your age. Any exercise that keeps your heart rate in the range of 65% - 75% of your maximum heart rate is optimal for fat burning and improving cardiovascular fitness. At least once during your daily aerobic activity, take your pulse. If you are below this range, you will need to step up the pace a bit. If you are too high, just slow down a little.

The Benefits of Strength Training

Strength training differs from aerobic training in three important ways. First, strength training involves activities that are more intense and much shorter in duration than aerobic activity, for example doing push-ups or sit-ups. Second, while aerobic training primarily improves the health of your cardiovascular system, strength training primarily improves the health of your muscles, bones and joints. Third, while aerobic activity should be performed almost every day for maximum benefit, you only need to engage in strength training two to three times per week. The benefits of strength training include:

- *Increased muscle and bone strength*
- *Improved muscle tone and body shape*
- *Improved hormone function*
- *Improved mood and mental functioning*
- *Decreased serum cholesterol*
- *Decreased stress*
- *More restful sleep*
- *Increased metabolism*
- *Prevent the muscle loss associated with dieting*

To benefit from strength training, it is not necessary that you spend long grueling hours in the gym every day. In fact, you can experience a significant improvement in your strength and muscle tone by weightlifting for one hour, two or three times a week!

The key to successful strength training is not the amount of time you spend; it's the intensity that is important. The harder you work your muscles during your strength workouts, the quicker you will see improvements.

How Your Muscle Responds to Strength Training

Your muscles do whatever you tell them to do. Strength training is simply a way to tell your muscles that you want them to get stronger. As long as you tell them often enough, they will begin to listen.

Each time you exercise your muscles hard, your body goes to work to build more muscle. As long as you continue to slowly increase the weight that you use week after week, your muscles will continue to grow in strength. Most people begin to see a difference in their strength and how they look after a few weeks of strength training.

There are a lot of misconceptions about strength training. Many people have heard myths such as if you stop lifting weights all of the muscle that you gained just turns to fat, or that strength training is not good for women.

Exercise Tips for the Very Large

Very large people face special challenges in trying to be active. You may not be able to bend or move in the same way that other people can. It may be hard to find clothes and equipment for exercising, and you may feel self-conscious being physically active around other people. Facing these challenges is hard, but it can be done.

When starting your exercise program, it is important to be easy on yourself. If you cannot do an activity, don't feel bad about it. Just feel good about what you can do and avoid negative self-talk. One very heavy woman once told me that if other people talked to her the way she sometimes talks to herself, she would punch them. Focus on the positive and you will improve your chances of success.

If you are a large person starting on an exercise program, it is important to start slowly. Your body needs time to get used to your new activity. Be sure to spend some time warming-up. Warm-ups get your body ready for action. Shrug your shoulders, tap your toes, swing your arms, or march in place. You should spend a few minutes warming up for any physical activity - even walking. Walk more slowly for the first few minutes.

Spend some time cooling-down. Slow down little by little. If you have been walking fast, walk slowly or stretch for a few minutes to cool down. Cooling down protects your heart, relaxes your muscles, and keeps you from getting hurt.

Most very large people can do some or all of the physical activities in this book, including:

- *Weight-bearing aerobic activities, like walking or using the elliptical machine, which involve lifting or pushing your own body weight.*
- *Non-weight-bearing aerobic activities, like swimming, water workouts and the exercise bicycle. These activities put less stress on your joints because you do not have to lift or push your own weight. If your feet or joints hurt when you stand, non-weight-bearing activities may be best for you.*
- *Strength training exercise. Most weightlifting exercises can be performed while seated or lying down. Strength training is the quickest and safest way for very large people to increase metabolism, improve strength and begin burning calories while minimizing the stress on the feet, knees and ankles.*

Be sure to pay attention to your body. If you are very large, your joints will carry much more weight than those who are leaner. If your feet, knees, or back begin to hurt from weight-bearing exercise, start out by doing non-weight-bearing exercises and slowly work up to doing weight-bearing exercises. Listening to your body will help you avoid potential injuries that could set you back.

If you are not active now, start slowly. Try to walk just 4 minutes per day for the first week. Walk 8 minutes per day the next week. Stay at 8–minute walks until you feel comfortable. Then increase your walks to 12 minutes. Slowly lengthen each walk by 4 minutes per week until you reach 20 minutes per day. Once you reach 20 minutes per day, you can work on quickening your pace to get your walking into the aerobic range. Please be patient! You will be much better off in the long run if you start slow and build slow.

You can do many activities in your home. There are some advantages to exercising in health clubs, however, including having access to a wider variety of exercise equipment and being around other people who can be a source of inspiration and support. You may feel self-conscious exercising around other people, but keep in mind that you have just as much right to be healthy and active as anyone. Even though you may feel like other people are judging you, they are not. In fact, most of the people who have the best physiques will be very supportive and they can be a great source of information.

The Dumbbell Row

The Dumbbell Row is without question the best overall upper back exercise you can do. It not only develops your rhomboid muscles very well, but it is also a powerful exercise to recoordinate all of the muscles of the upper and mid-back. It also improves the motion in the entire back and encourages proper posture.

Although this is not a difficult exercise to do, many people find it difficult at first because their upper back muscles are not coordinated. If the Dumbbell Row is done correctly, you should feel the muscles between your shoulder blades getting a good workout. But don't be alarmed if you don't feel anything at first or if you feel it more in your arms. As the muscles in your upper back begin to fire correctly, you should feel the muscles between your shoulder blades working.

To do the Dumbbell Row, place one hand on the seat of your chair and hold a dumbbell in the other. Most people find it comfortable to step back with the outside foot as shown in the picture. Keep your back straight, keep the palm of your dumbbell hand facing toward your legs and allow the dumbbell to hang toward the floor.

Keeping your back straight and your face toward the floor, raise your elbow out to the side and point it toward the ceiling, allowing your upper back to twist so that the dumbbell lightly touches your shoulder. Once the weight has touched your shoulder, gently lower it back down. One repetition should take four to five seconds.

The Dumbbell Row

Benefits: Upper Back Strength

Equipment Needed: Pair of Dumbbells, Chair

Time / Repetitions: 10-15 Repetitions

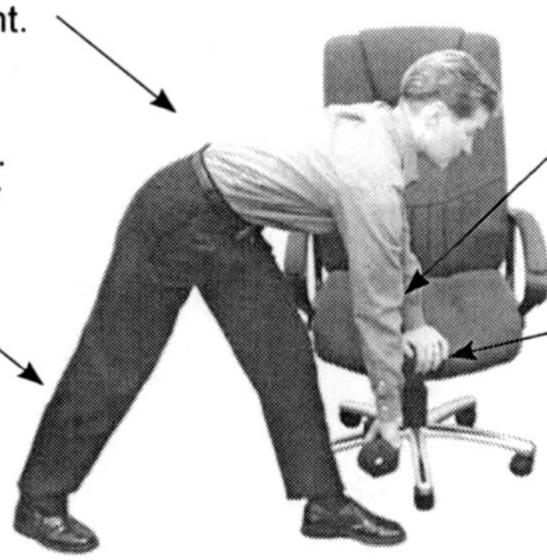

Step 1:

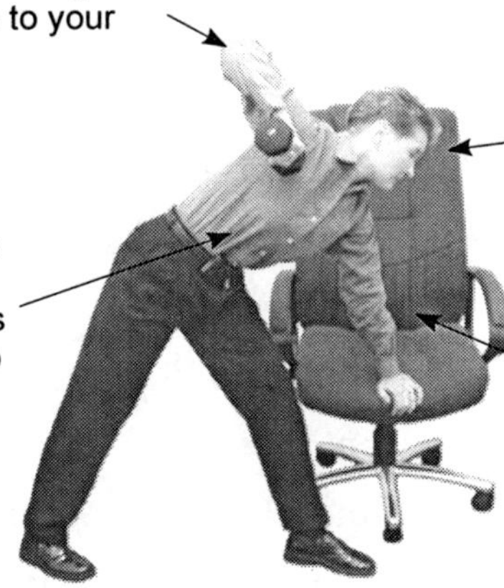
Point your elbow toward the ceiling while lifting the dumbbell up to your shoulder.
Keep your eyes focused on the floor.
Allow your torso to twist so that your chest faces perpendicular to the floor.
Keep your elbow straight.

Step 2:

The Dumbbell Shrug

The Dumbbell Shrug is a great exercise for the trapezius muscle, especially the upper portion of the muscle which runs from the base of the neck, up to the base of the skull and out to the shoulders. Most people who work at desk jobs have a lot of tightness and pain in this area. The Dumbbell Shrug will help to relax the trapezius, increase circulation and decrease the "knots" in the muscle.

To do the Dumbbell Shrug, stand up straight with a dumbbell in each hand. Draw your shoulders back so that your shoulder blades squeeze together while raising your shoulders as high as you can toward your ears. Then gently let the weights back down again. Each repetition should take four to five seconds to complete.

The trapezius is considerably stronger than the rhomboid muscle. Consequently, you will be able to lift much more weight doing the Dumbbell Shrug than the Dumbbell Row. However, in order to achieve proper muscle balance in the upper back, I encourage you to use the same weight for both exercises. Here's why: in most people the trapezius is tight, inflamed and full of trigger points and already too strong in comparison to the rhomboid muscle. The goal of exercising the trapezius should not be to make it stronger but rather to improve blood flow and to decrease the amount of muscle tension. This can be accomplished by exercising the trapezius with a light weight while building strength in the rhomboids.

The Dumbbell Shrug

Benefits:	Upper Back and Neck Strength
Equipment Needed:	Pair of Dumbbells
Time / Repetitions:	10-15 Repetitions

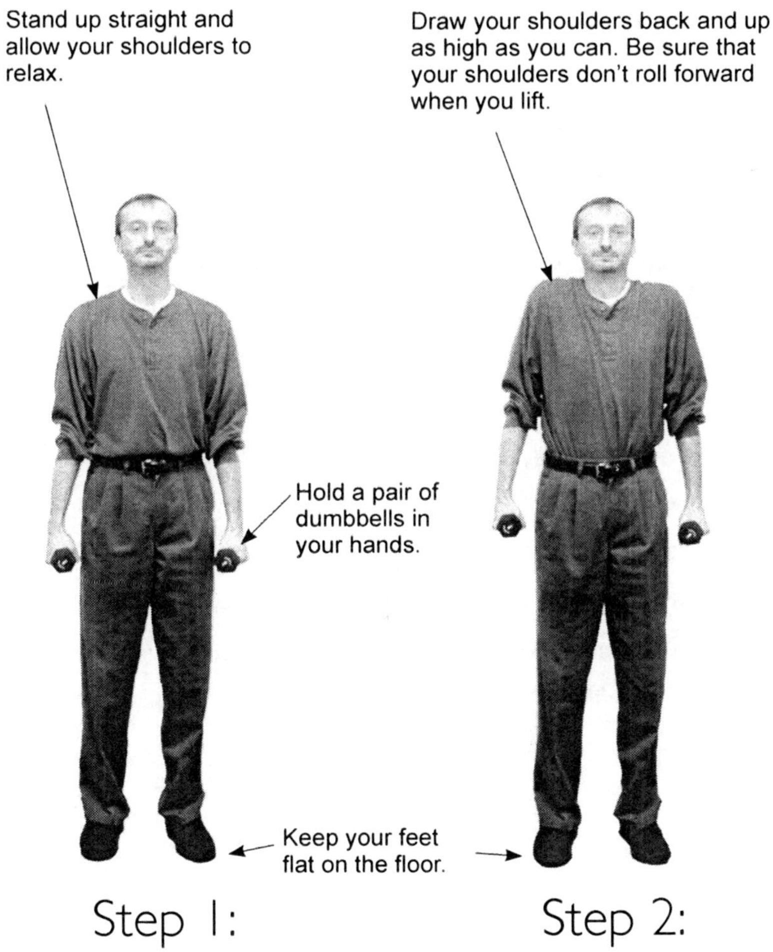

The Opening Stretch

This is a great stretch to help alleviate tension in the upper back and neck. Best of all, it only takes 30 seconds and you don't even have to get out of your chair.

To begin the Opening Stretch, scoot forward in your chair so that you are sitting comfortably on the front portion of your seat. Sit up nice and straight with both feet flat on the floor. With your upper arms hanging down to your side, bend your elbows 90 degrees and turn your palms upward so that they face toward the ceiling.

Now slowly rotate your hands outward, keeping your elbows against your torso, so that you feel a nice squeeze between the shoulder blades. Turn your feet outward as far as you can. Tip your head back slightly to remove the tension from your neck muscles, and if you'd like, close your eyes. Take three deep, slow breaths, allowing ten seconds for each breath. Just count to yourself as you breathe in "one, two, three, four, five" and back out again "six, seven, eight, nine, ten."

Many people find it beneficial to do this exercise several times during the workday, especially people who do a lot of work on a computer.

The Opening Stretch

Benefits:	Upper Back and Neck Strength
Equipment Needed:	Chair
Time / Repetitions:	30 Seconds

Step 1:

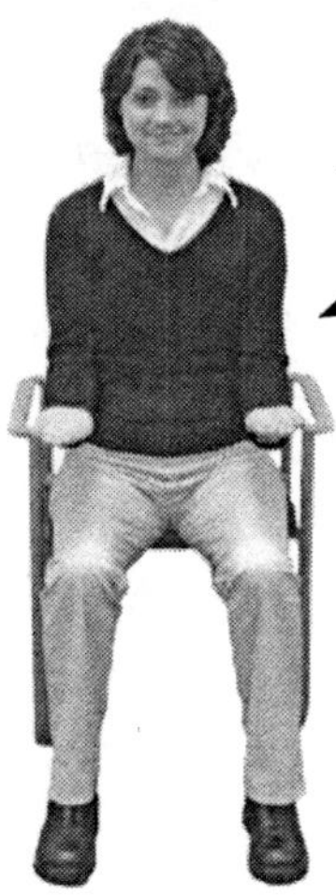

Sit up straight and slide to the front edge of your chair.

Bend your elbows 90 degrees and hold them against your side.

Turn your palms upward.

Step 2:

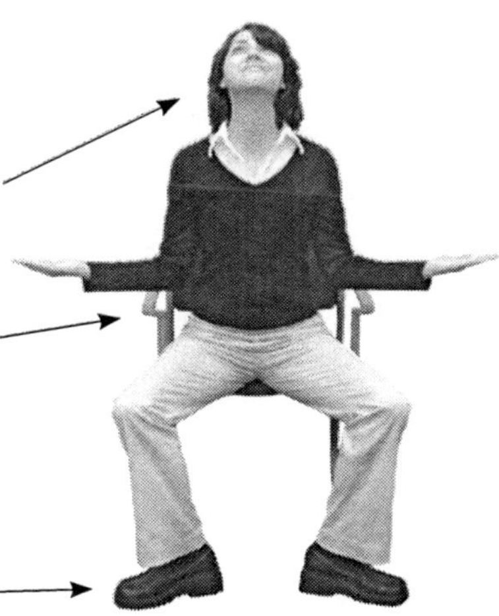

Tilt your head back and take three deep breaths.

Keeping your elbows locked to your side, rotate your hands out as far as you can.

Turn your feet outward.

The Upper Back Stretch

The Upper Back Stretch is great for improving the overall mobility and flexibility in your upper back. A very common problem with working at a desk job is that your upper back does not have the opportunity to move very much. Consequently, the joints in your spine get "sticky" and your muscles shorten. This stretch helps to keep your joints and the muscles in your upper back nice and loose.

To do the Upper Back Stretch, start by sitting up straight in your chair. Take your right hand and place it on the outside of your left knee. Twist your torso toward the left while rounding your upper back until you feel a stretch between your shoulder blades in your upper back as shown on the opposite page. Hold this position for 15 seconds, then do the Upper Back Stretch again to the opposite side.

The Upper Back Stretch

Benefits: Upper Back Flexibility

Equipment Needed: Chair

Time / Repetitions: 15 Seconds on Each Side

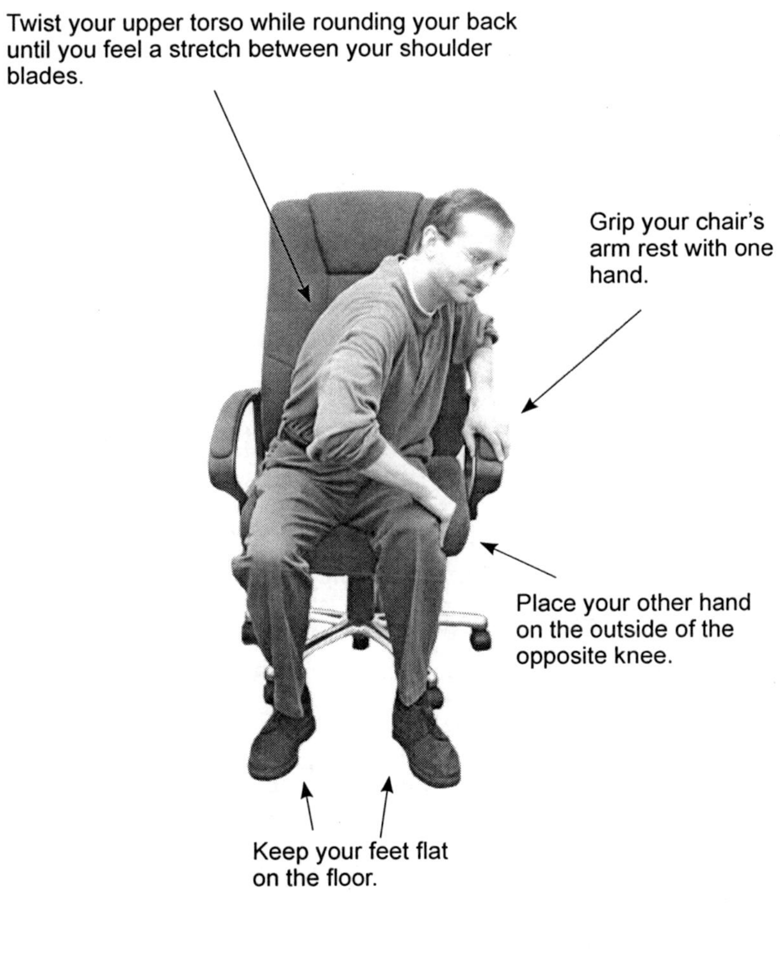

Neck Rolls

This simple exercise is designed to improve mobility in the neck. To do this exercise, scoot up to the front part of your seat and sit up nice and straight. Slowly let your head drop forward and let your chin drop to your chest. From that position slowly rotate your head until your right ear is resting close to your right shoulder. Then, slowly rotate your head back so that your head is tipped back as far as is comfortable. Finally, rotate your head to the left side until your left ear is resting close to your left shoulder.

It is important that you do this exercise slowly and you do not try to force your neck further than it can move comfortably. It is also important to keep your shoulders down while doing Neck Rolls. You can hold the bottom of your seat with both hands if you need help keeping your shoulders down.

Don't be surprised if you hear some crackling in your neck when you perform Neck Rolls. Usually this crackling, also called "crepitus," may go away after doing this exercise for a while, and it poses no hazard. If the crepitus does not go away, it may indicate that there is some scar tissue that has formed in the joint cartilage. Although the crackling may be annoying, it shouldn't be a cause for concern.

If you notice that your neck won't roll as well on one side as it will on the other, there may be some vertebrae that are stuck. This requires chiropractic care in order to help these vertebrae function correctly again.

Neck Rolls

Benefits:	Neck Mobility
Equipment Needed:	Chair
Time / Repetitions:	15 Rotations in Each Direction

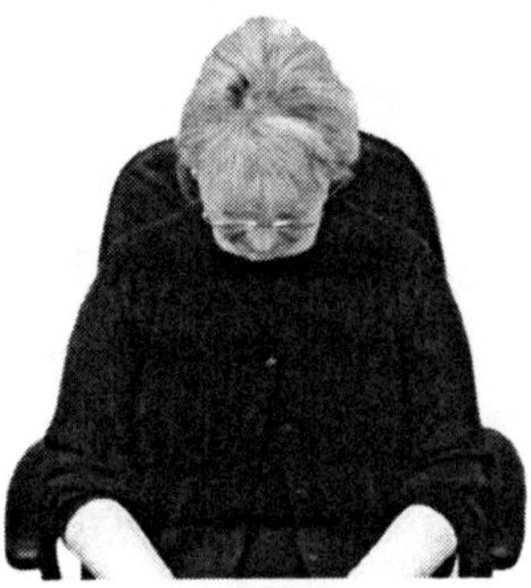

Step 1:

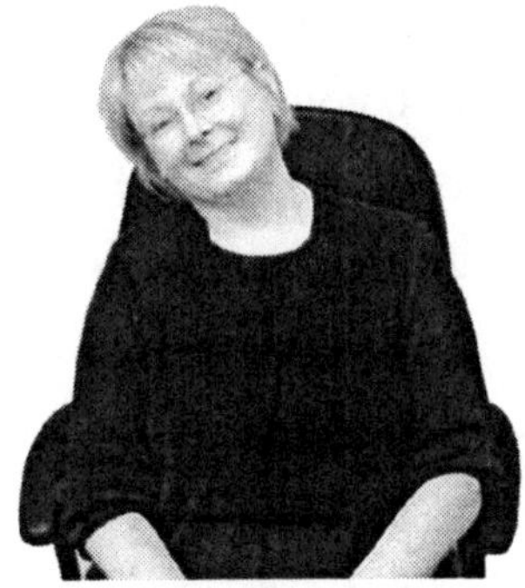

Step 2:

When doing Neck Rolls, it is important to do three things in order to properly stretch the muscles of the neck: 1) keep your shoulders perfectly level, 2) keep your face oriented forward, and 3) roll your head slowly. It should take 30 seconds to make one complete revolution.

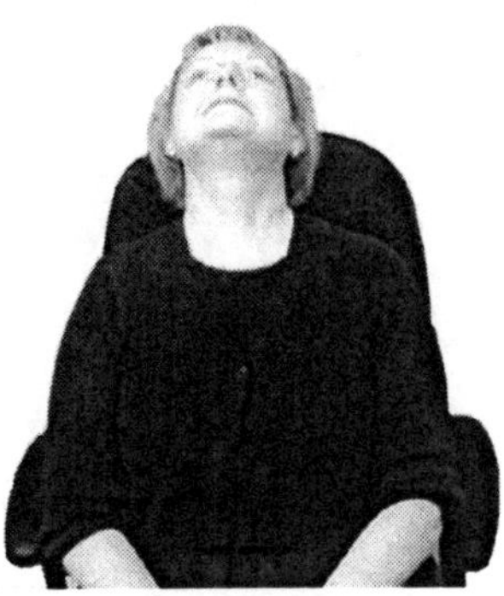

Step 3:

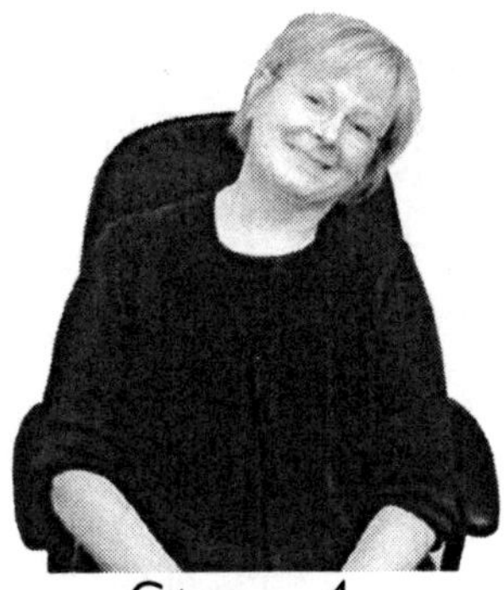

Step 4:

The Chair Neck Stretch

The Chair Neck Stretch can be used to decrease the tightness of the trapezius and levator scapulae, as well as the scalene muscles. To do the Chair Neck Stretch, scoot up to the front edge of your chair and sit up straight. With your right hand, grasp the bottom of the seat of your chair. Reach over the top of your head with your left hand and place it on the right side of your head. Gently lean toward the left while tipping your head to the left until you feel a good stretch in the neck and shoulder muscles. Hold this stretch for 30-45 seconds, then switch sides.

You can vary the muscles stretched by placing your hand on different parts of your chair seat and leaning your head at different angles. To stretch primarily your trapezius and levator scapulae, grip your seat just behind your hip and tilt your head slightly forward and to the side. To stretch primarily your scalenes, grip your seat at about your mid-thigh and tilt your head slightly backward and to the side. Remember that the muscles of the neck are small and somewhat fragile, so stretch gently and hold without bouncing.

The Chair Neck Stretch

Benefits:	Neck Mobility
Equipment Needed:	Chair
Time / Repetitions:	30-40 Seconds on Each Side

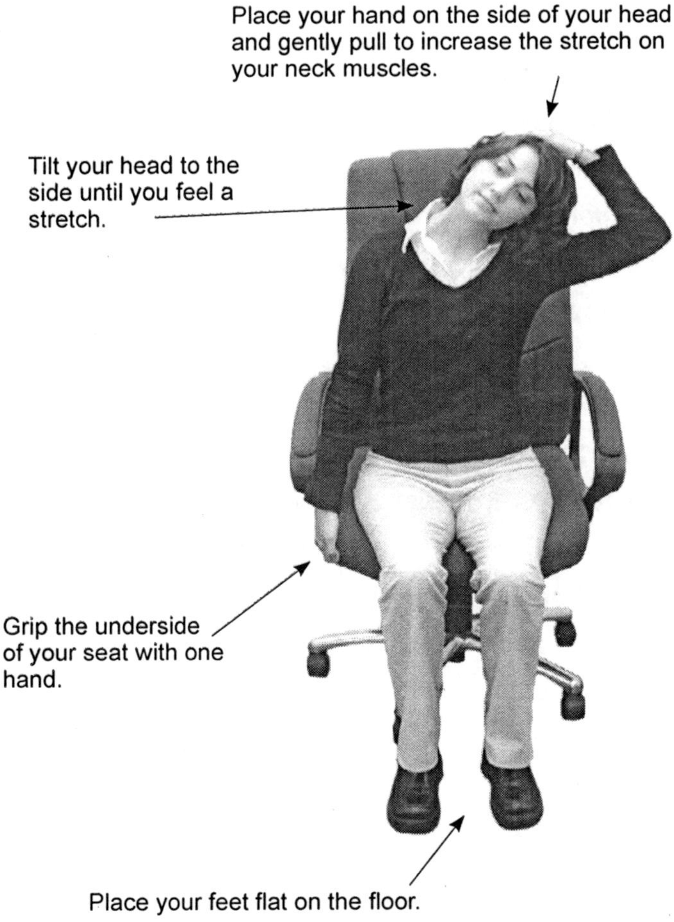

The Wall Posture

This simple exercise is designed to directly counteract the unhealthy neck and upper back posture found in people who work at desk jobs; namely, the head being carried too far forward and the hunching of the upper back.

To do this exercise, simply stand up against a wall, making sure that your heels, pelvis, shoulders and the back of your head are all touching the wall. Make sure that your head stays level and that you glide your head backward, rather than tilting your head back in order to touch the wall with your head. This will require you to pull your chin down toward your chest a bit.

Once you have successfully positioned yourself into this Wall Posture, slowly step away from the wall and go about your business while holding the posture as long as possible. If you have done this correctly, it will probably feel somewhat unusual to walk around like this. But don't worry, you don't look as funny as you feel. As a matter of fact, to everyone else, you probably look better. People with good posture look better than those with bad posture.

It is important that you try to hold this posture while you go back about your business in order to retrain your body mechanics. For this reason, most people find it necessary to do this exercise several times throughout the day as a checkup on their posture.

The Wall Posture

Benefits: Neck and Upper Back Posture

Equipment Needed: Wall

Time / Repetitions: Maintain as Long as Possible

Stand up against a wall so that your shoulders, hips and heels are all touching the wall.

Keeping your head level, draw your neck back until the back of your head touches the wall.

Step away from the wall while maintaining this new head posture. Keep this head posture as long as you can while you work.

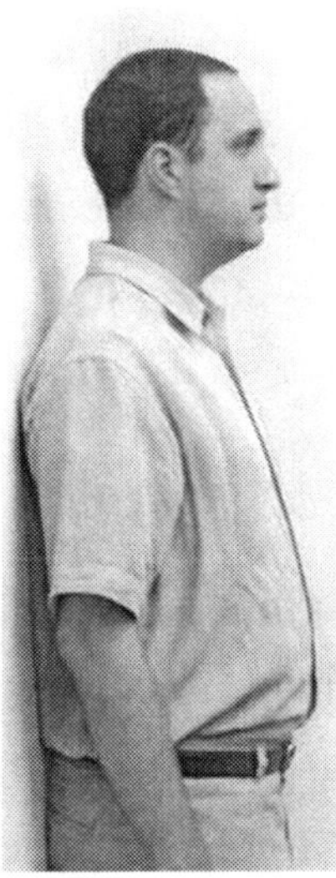

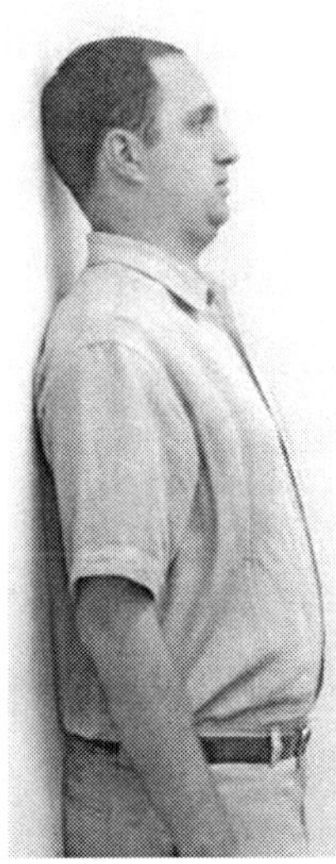

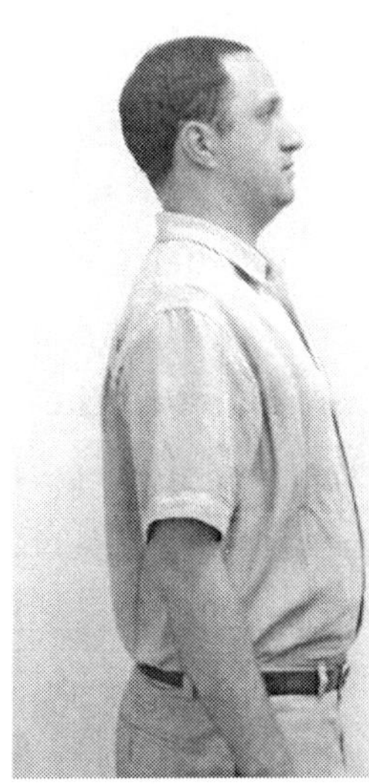

Step 1: Step 2:Step 3:

Stiff-Leg Deadlifts

With the exception of abdominal muscle strengthening, the Stiff-Leg Deadlift is the single-most important exercise to strengthen and recoordinate all of the muscles of the low back and pelvis. To do this exercise, you will want to start by standing up straight with your feet about shoulder width apart, a pair of dumbbells in your hands and your knees bent slightly—about 10-15 degrees. The object is to bend forward at the hips, allowing the dumbbells to drop just below the knees and then to straighten back up again, all the while keeping your head up, your back straight, and your knees bent slightly.

It is very important when bending at the hips that you do not cheat and bend at the waist. If you do this exercise correctly, you should feel most of the exercise in your hamstrings rather than in your low back. If you feel it mostly in your low back, it means that you are not pushing your hips back far enough and that you are bending at the waist. Many people find it helpful to imagine that they are carefully sitting down on a chair behind them while keeping their back straight.

You will want each repetition of lowering the weights down and lifting them back up to take approximately six to eight seconds. One other thing about the Stiff-Leg Deadlifts: since you are working large muscles, you will want to use dumbbells that are heavy enough to challenge the muscles; 15-25 pound dumbbells are probably a good place to start.

Stiff-Leg Deadlifts

Benefits:	Low Back Strength and Coordination
Equipment Needed:	Pair of Dumbbells
Time / Repetitions:	10-15 Repetitions

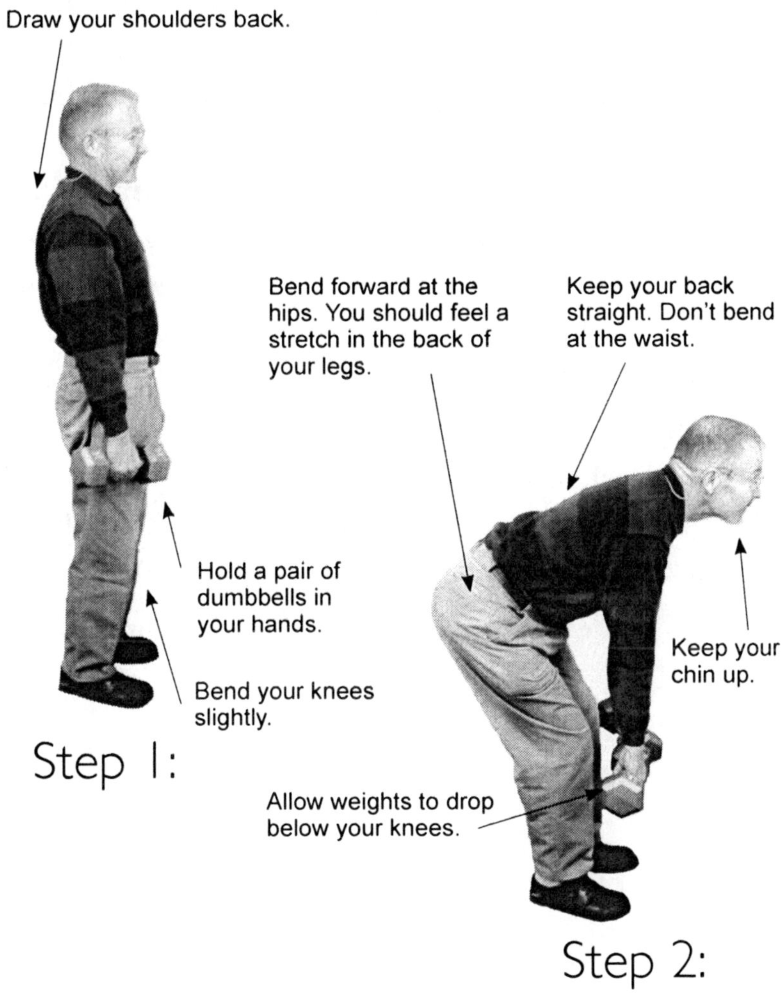
Draw your shoulders back.
Hold a pair of dumbbells in your hands.
Bend your knees slightly.
Step 1:
Bend forward at the hips. You should feel a stretch in the back of your legs.
Keep your back straight. Don't bend at the waist.
Keep your chin up.
Allow weights to drop below your knees.
Step 2:

Pelvic Tilts

Pelvic Tilts are one of the easiest exercises to help increase abdominal strength. To do this exercise, stand up straight and place your hands on your hips. Exhale completely while contracting your abdominal muscles and tilting your pelvis as shown in the picture on the opposite page. Hold this position for three seconds, then inhale and allow your body to return to the starting position. Each repetition should take approximately three to five seconds.

Depending on the condition of your body when you begin doing Pelvic Tilts, you may feel your abdominals getting a good workout from this exercise, but don't be discouraged if you do not feel this at first.

You can make this exercise even more intense by drawing your abdomen in as far as you can after you completely exhale. You should feel a contraction in your oblique muscles just to the side of your abdominals. This extra contraction of the obliques helps to flatten the belly.

Pelvic Tilts

Benefits:	Abdominal Strength
Equipment Needed:	None
Time / Repetitions:	As Many as Possible

Step 1:

Step 2:

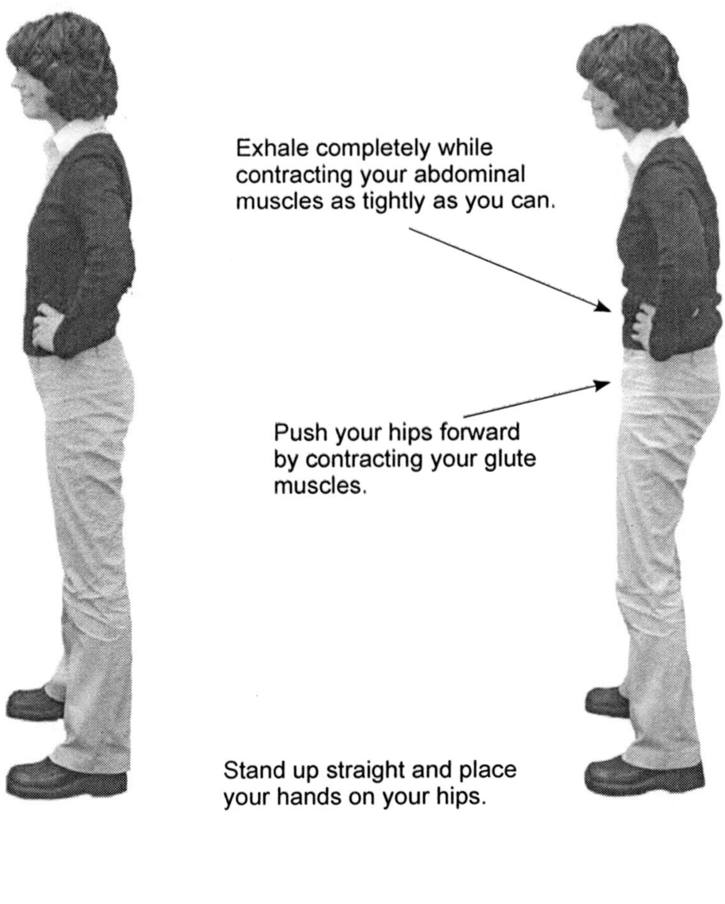

Chair Crunches

Chair Crunches are designed to help increase abdominal strength while improving balance and coordination. To do this exercise, scoot forward in the seat of your chair so that your buttocks rest on the front edge of the seat but the backs of your legs are not touching the chair. Keeping your back straight, lean back slightly and grip the armrests of your chair with both hands. Using your abdominal muscles, raise your knees as far toward your chest as you can. Hold this position for one second and then slowly lower your knees back down. Each repetition should take approximately three to four seconds.

You can decrease the difficulty of this exercise by keeping your knees bent so that your feet stay close to your body. The more you straighten your legs, the more difficult this exercise becomes.

Depending on the condition of your body when you begin doing Chair Crunches, you may feel your abdominals getting a good workout from this exercise, but don't be discouraged if you do not feel this at first. Initially, you may feel it more in your low back or even legs. This is common when the abdominal muscles have lost their natural coordination. Just keep at it and soon your abdominal muscles will come around.

Chair Crunches

Benefits: Abdominal Strength

Equipment Needed: Chair

Time / Repetitions: As Many as Possible Without Pain

Step 1:

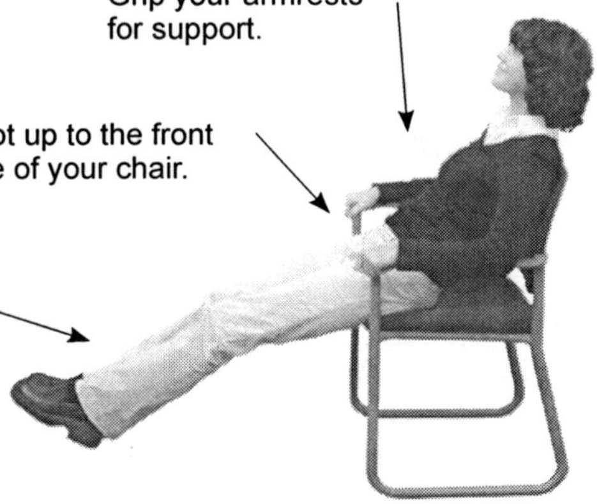

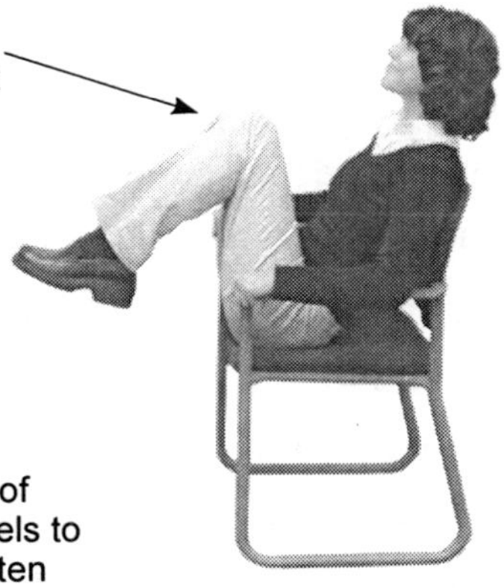

Note: You can increase the intensity of this exercise by not allowing your heels to touch the floor each time you straighten your legs.

Step 2:

The Cobra Stretch

The Cobra Stretch is great for improving the flexibility of the abdominal and psoas muscles as well as increasing mobility in the low back. When doing this exercise, be sure that your chair is pushed up against a wall so that it doesn't move away from you. To do the Cobra Stretch, stand facing your chair, with your feet shoulder width apart and about 24"-36" away from the edge of your chair. Lean forward and grip the center of your armrests. Keeping your arms straight, allow your pelvis to drop toward the seat of your chair and lift your chin toward the ceiling. You should feel a considerable stretch in the abdominals when you do this stretch correctly.

You can adjust the intensity of the stretch by how far you place your feet from your chair. The farther away your feet are, the more intense the stretch will be on your abdominal muscles.

Depending on the strength of your upper body, you may find it difficult to support your weight with your arms for very long. If this happens, you can step forward with your feet slightly to decrease the weight supported by the arms and make sure that you keep your elbows straight. After a few weeks of doing this stretch, your arms will become stronger and it will be easier to support yourself.

Discontinue doing this stretch if you feel pain in your low back and just stick with the other low back exercises and stretches for a couple of weeks before trying this stretch again. As your back becomes healthier, you should be able to do this stretch without experiencing back pain.

The Cobra Stretch

Benefits:	Flexibility in the Low Back
Equipment Needed:	Chair
Time / Repetitions:	30-45 Seconds

Step 1:

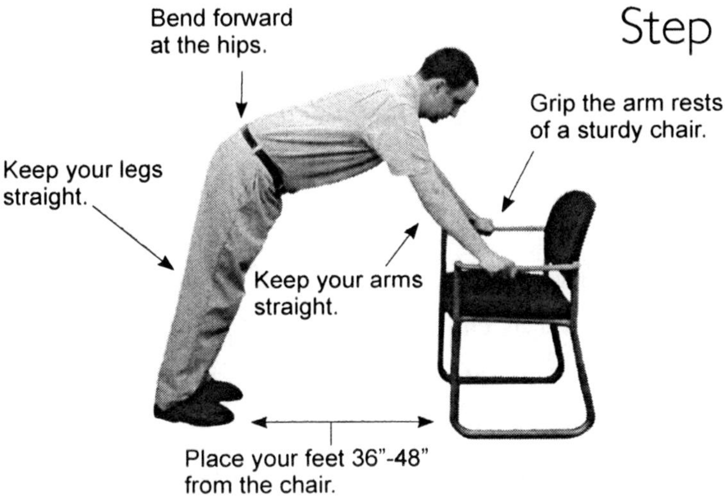

Bend forward at the hips.
Grip the arm rests of a sturdy chair.
Keep your legs straight.
Keep your arms straight.
Place your feet 36"-48" from the chair.

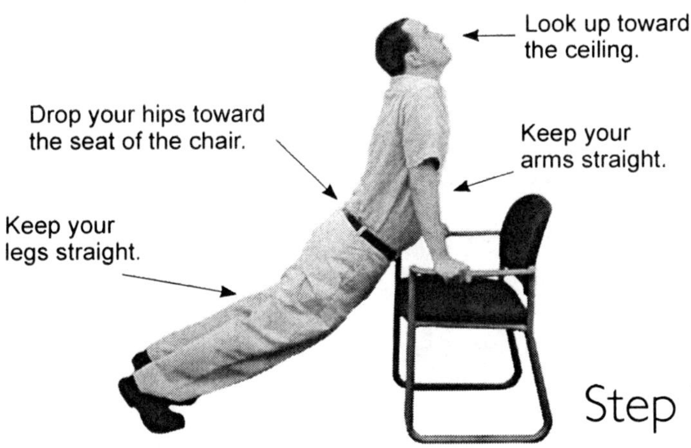

Step 2:

The Chair Low Back Stretch

This stretch is a quick way to reduce tension in the low back and is perfect for a mini-break during the day. To do this stretch, scoot forward to the front part of your seat and straighten your legs. Allowing your spine to bend forward, reach your hands as far down the front of your legs as possible and allow your head to drop toward your thighs. Take slow, deep breaths for 30-45 seconds, then sit back up again.

If you have a difficult time getting your low back to bend forward, which many people do, it could be for a couple of reasons. The first is that if your hamstring muscles are too tight, they will hold your pelvis in place and not allow it to roll forward. If your pelvis cannot roll forward, your low back will not be able to bend as far forward. If this is the case with you, doing hamstring stretches will help.

The other reason why you may not be able roll your back forward is that the joints in your low back are stuck and are not allowing the vertebrae to move correctly. This is very common among people who work at desk jobs. The only way to get the joints in the low back moving correctly again is through chiropractic care. If this stretch is difficult for you, it is a good idea to have your low back checked out by a chiropractor.

The Chair Low Back Stretch

Benefits:	Decrease Tension in the Low Back
Equipment Needed:	Chair
Time / Repetitions:	30-45 Seconds

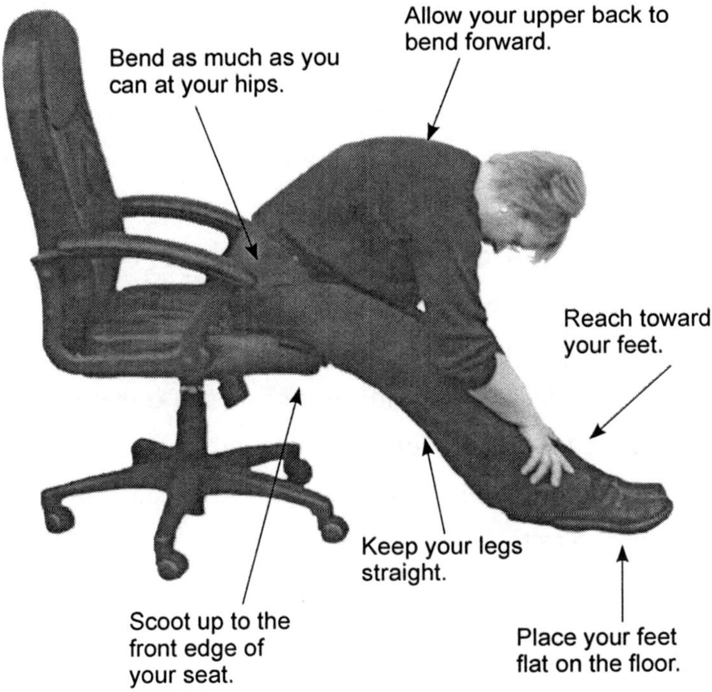
Allow your upper back to bend forward.
Bend as much as you can at your hips.
Reach toward your feet.
Keep your legs straight.
Scoot up to the front edge of your seat.
Place your feet flat on the floor.

The Glute Medius Stretch

The Glute Medius Stretch is very effective in reducing the stress in the hip and buttock area. To do this stretch, scoot up to the front part of your seat and rest the ankle of one leg on the thigh of the other. Sit up nice and straight and place both hands around the knee of your topmost leg, interlacing your fingers. Using a gentle pull, draw your knee up to the opposite shoulder and hold the position for 30-45 seconds. Then switch legs and do the same stretch to the other leg. If you do this stretch correctly, you should feel a good stretch in the buttock.

This stretch is very important for people who sit a lot at work because the muscles in the buttocks and pelvis become very tight. This tightness contributes to pain and loss of flexibility in the low back.

If you find that you don't have enough flexibility to cross your legs as pictured, you can start by gripping one knee with both of your hands and pulling your knee toward your chest and holding the stretch for 30-45 seconds. Over time, the glute medius and piriformis muscles will relax and allow you to perform the stretch as shown.

The Glute Medius Stretch

Benefits:	Pelvis and Hip Flexibility
Equipment Needed:	Chair
Time / Repetitions:	30-45 Seconds on Each Side

Step 1:

Sit up straight in your chair.

Cross one leg over the other and grab your knee with both hands.

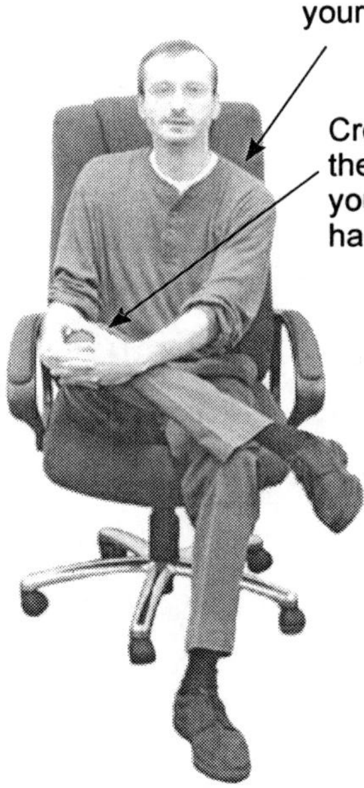

Step 2:

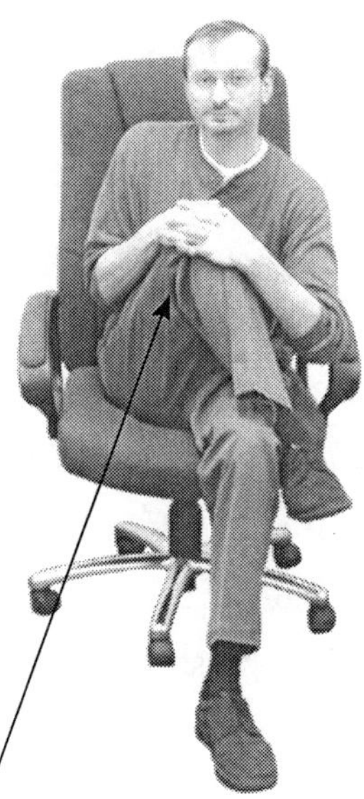

Keeping your back straight, pull your knee up as high up toward the opposite shoulder as you can. Hold the stretch for 30-45 seconds.

The Psoas Stretch

A tight psoas muscle is one of the biggest contributors to the low back pain experienced by most people who sit at work. This stretch is designed to decrease the tension in the psoas muscle and improve the mobility and flexibility in the low back. To do this stretch, start with both feet together, your back straight and one of your hands resting on your chair or a wall for balance. Take a large step back with one of your legs as shown in the picture on the opposite page. Keeping your back leg straight and allowing your front leg to bend at the knee, push the hip of your back leg forward until you feel a stretch in the upper inside front part of the thigh. Hold this stretch for 30-45 seconds, then switch legs.

The key to doing this stretch is keeping the hips in the correct position. If you do not feel a stretch in the right place, it is likely that you are allowing your hips to turn to the side and are not keeping them facing the front. The other thing that could be happening is that you may be trying to keep your back foot flat on the floor. In order for the back leg to have enough mobility to stretch the psoas muscle, it will be necessary to raise your heel.

If you have good balance, you can increase the intensity of the stretch by raising your hands above your head and tipping your upper body backwards slightly while looking at the ceiling. This offers you the added benefit of stretching the abdominal muscles at the same time.

The Psoas Stretch

Benefits:	Low Back and Pelvis Flexibility
Equipment Needed:	None
Time / Repetitions:	30-45 Seconds on Each Side

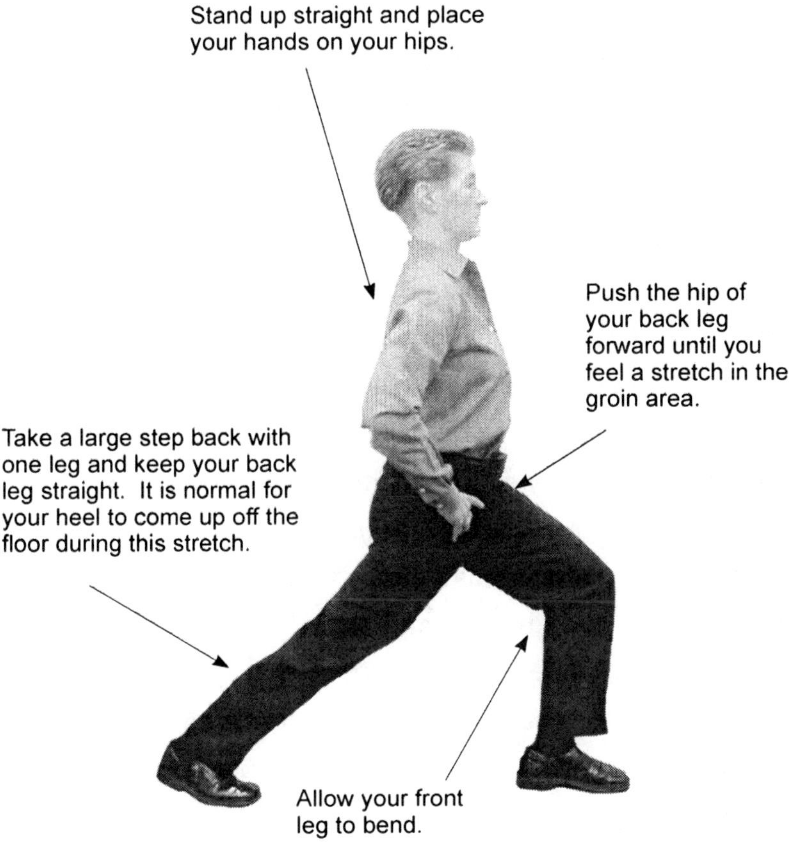
Stand up straight and place your hands on your hips.
Push the hip of your back leg forward until you feel a stretch in the groin area.
Take a large step back with one leg and keep your back leg straight. It is normal for your heel to come up off the floor during this stretch.
Allow your front leg to bend.

The Lunge

You can do Lunges with or without weights depending on your physical condition. If you have not done Lunges before, I suggest that you start without weights. To do the Lunge, start with your feet together and one hand resting on the back of a chair for balance. Step back with one leg so that your legs are about 60 degrees apart. Keeping your back straight, allow your knees to bend until you touch the floor with the knee of your back leg, then straighten your legs again. Repeat this exercise 10-15 times for each leg.

If you have knee problems, you may have to modify the Lunge somewhat to make it easier on your knees. One way of doing this is to place a phone book or two on the floor in front of your back leg so that your back knee only drops to within six inches from the floor. If this is still too stressful for your knees, just go down as far as you can. The further down you can go, the better, as long as it doesn't strain your knees.

This is a great exercise to improve the strength and flexibility in the quadriceps and glute muscles as well as to improve your overall coordination and sense of balance. After doing Lunges for a while, you will notice that it is easier to climb stairs, easier to squat down to grab something off of the floor, and that there will be less soreness in your buttocks and legs from prolonged sitting.

The Lunge

Benefits:	Quadriceps and Glute Strength
Equipment Needed:	Chair
Time / Repetitions:	10-15 Repetitions for Each Leg

Step 1:

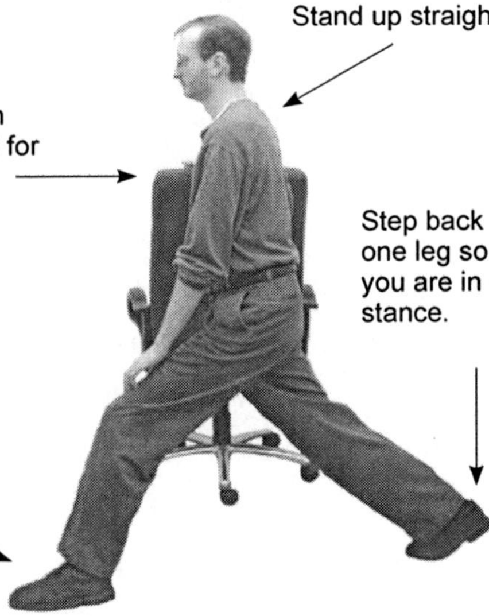
Stand up straight.
Place your hand on your chair or a wall for balance.
Step back with one leg so that you are in a wide stance.
Your front foot should remain stationary during the exercise.

Step 2:

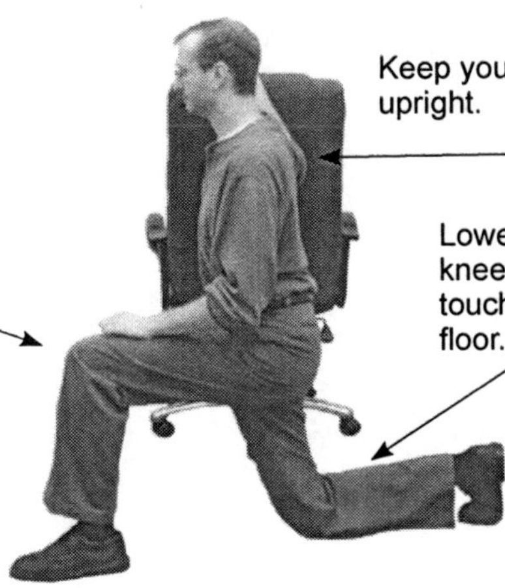

Calf Raises

Calf Raises are great for improving the strength and flexibility of your calf muscles. To do Calf Raises you will need a phone book or a stair step. Begin by placing the ball of your foot on the edge of the step or phone book so that your heel hangs freely in the air. Slowly lower your heel as far as you can, then raise your heel up as high as you can and hold this for one second. You will probably have to place your hand on the back of your chair or on a wall to maintain your balance when doing this exercise. Repeat this exercise 20-30 times.

One of the problems with a desk job is that most people begin to suffer the effects from decreased circulation in the legs. The veins in your legs require the exercise of the leg muscles in order to move your blood back to your heart effectively. When this does not happen, you can develop varicose and spider veins as well as swelling around the ankles.

The leg exercises in this section will go a long way to counteracting the decreased circulation in the legs, which is associated with sitting.

Calf Raises

Benefits:	Calf Strength
Equipment Needed:	Stair Step or Phone Book
Time / Repetitions:	20-30 Repetitions

Note: When doing Calf Raises, you will want to place your hand on a chair or a wall to help maintain your balance.

Place the ball of your foot at the edge of the phone book, allowing your heels to hang over the edge.

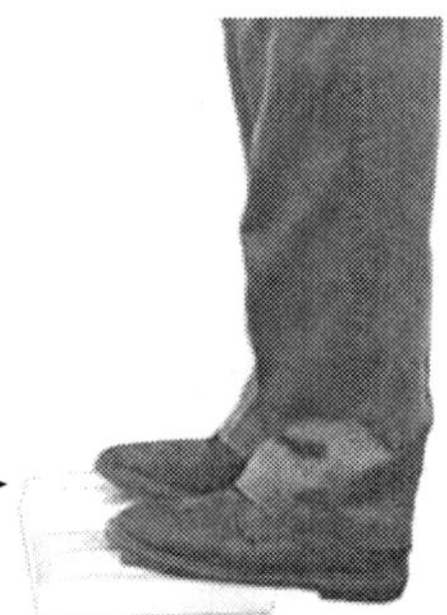

Step 1:

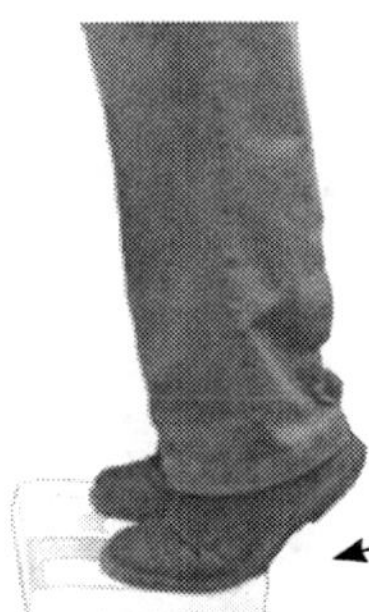

Lift your heels up as high as you can and hold them in this position for one second before lowering them back to the floor.

Step 2:

As an alternative, you can do this exercise on a stair step or any other object that is at least two inches high. To make this exercise a bit more challenging, try doing this exercise using only one leg at a time.

The Quadriceps Stretch

The Quadriceps Stretch is a great way to reduce the tension and improve the flexibility in the front of the thigh. To do the Quadriceps Stretch, start by standing next to chair or a wall and placing your hand on it for balance. Raise one foot backwards by bending your knee and grasping the foot with your free hand. Gently pull your leg back and press your foot against your buttock until you feel a stretch in the front part of your thigh. Hold this position for 30-45 seconds, then slowly release your hand from your foot and allow your foot to drop back to the floor. Repeat this stretch on the opposite leg.

Since the quadriceps are such big muscle groups, you will notice an immediate decrease in your overall tension level just by doing this stretch. This maneuver along with the next two stretches for the hamstrings and the calves should be done at least once a day for maximum benefit. I recommend doing each of these stretches twice per day, once early and once in the later part of the day.

The Quadriceps Stretch

Benefits:	Quadriceps Flexibility
Equipment Needed:	None
Time / Repetitions:	30-45 Seconds on Each Side

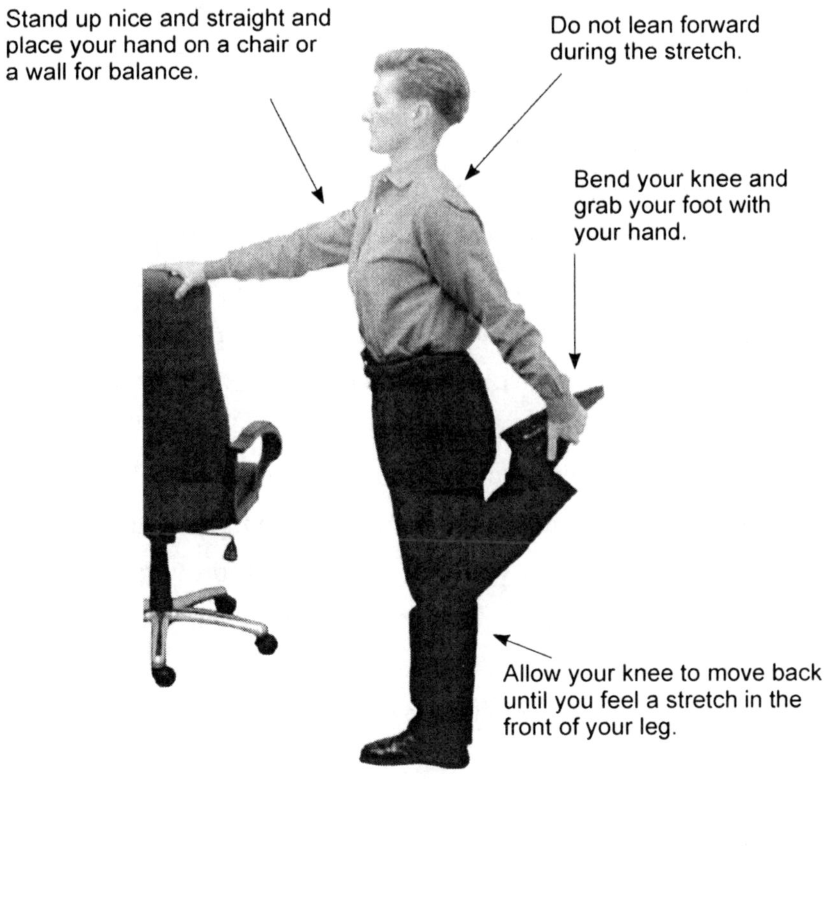
Stand up nice and straight and place your hand on a chair or a wall for balance.
Do not lean forward during the stretch.
Bend your knee and grab your foot with your hand.
Allow your knee to move back until you feel a stretch in the front of your leg.

The Triangle Stretch

The Triangle Stretch is great for improving the flexibility of the hamstrings and adductors. To do this stretch, start by facing your chair; place both hands on the arm rests and place your feet as far apart as you comfortably can. Slowly bend at the hips so that your pelvis drops back behind your feet and your body drops toward the seat of your chair. You should feel a good stretch in your hamstrings, as well as in the inside part of your upper leg. Hold this stretch for 30-45 seconds without bouncing.

If you don't feel a stretch in the back of your legs, you may be doing one of three things incorrectly. First, you may have your feet too far away from the chair; try moving your feet a little closer. Second, you may not have your feet spread far enough; try moving them a little farther apart. Third, you may be bending at the waist instead of at the hips; try bending more at the hips as in the Stiff-Leg Deadlifts.

The Triangle Stretch is a must for people with desk jobs, as prolonged sitting causes the hamstrings to tighten up. If you do this stretch regularly, you will notice an improvement in your flexibility, you will be more comfortable when you have to sit for long periods, and it will even decrease the stress on your low back, helping to reduce back pain.

The Triangle Stretch

Benefits: Hamstrings and Adductor Flexibility

Equipment Needed: Chair

Time / Repetitions: 30-45 Seconds

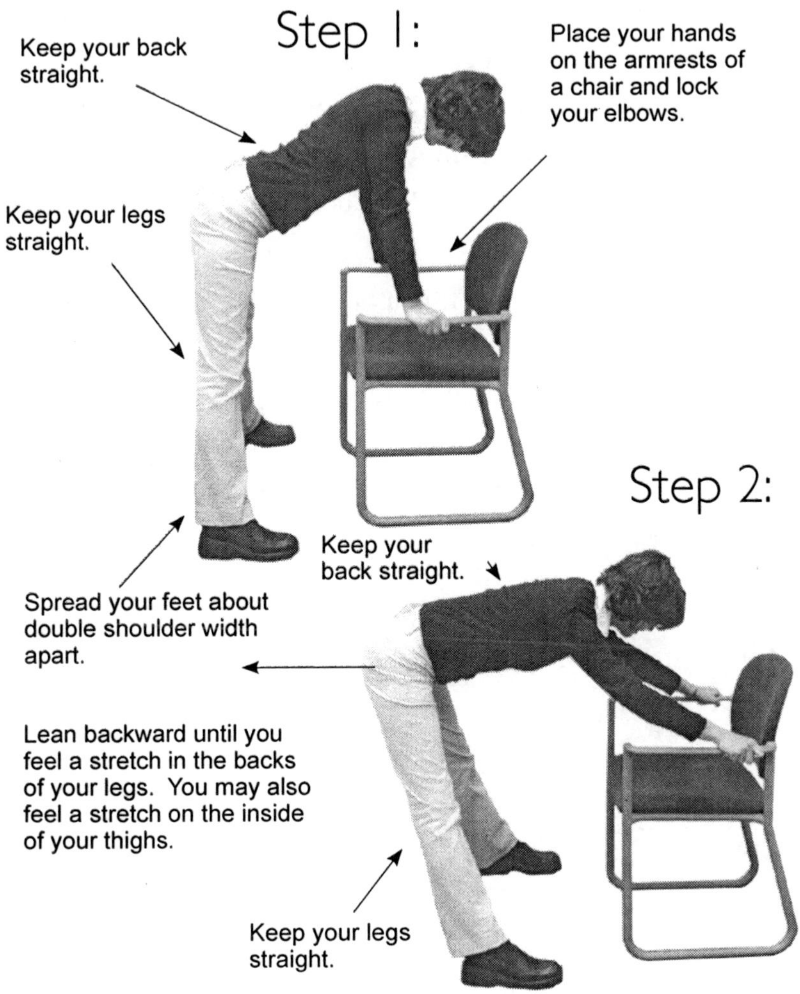
Step 1:
Keep your back straight.
Place your hands on the armrests of a chair and lock your elbows.
Keep your legs straight.
Spread your feet about double shoulder width apart.
Step 2:
Keep your back straight.
Lean backward until you feel a stretch in the backs of your legs. You may also feel a stretch on the inside of your thighs.
Keep your legs straight.

The Calf Stretch

The Calf Stretch is one of three important stretches, along with the Triangle Stretch and the Quadriceps Stretch, that will keep your legs flexible and relaxed during a long day at work. To do this stretch, start by facing a wall approximately an arm's length away. Place both hands on the wall and take a big step back with one of your legs, allowing the leg closest to the wall to bend at the knee. Gently allow your back heel to drop toward the floor until you feel a stretch in your calf muscles. Hold this stretch for 30-45 seconds without bouncing, then switch legs.

As you read in the Calf Raises exercise description, the calf muscles are not only responsible for walking, but they also help with pumping blood back to the heart. When the calf muscles, and to some degree the hamstrings, are chronically tight and don't get enough exercise, blood tends to pool in the lower legs and can lead to painful varicose veins and swelling in the ankles.

The Calf Stretch

Benefits:	Calf Flexibility
Equipment Needed:	Wall
Time / Repetitions:	30-45 Seconds on Each Side

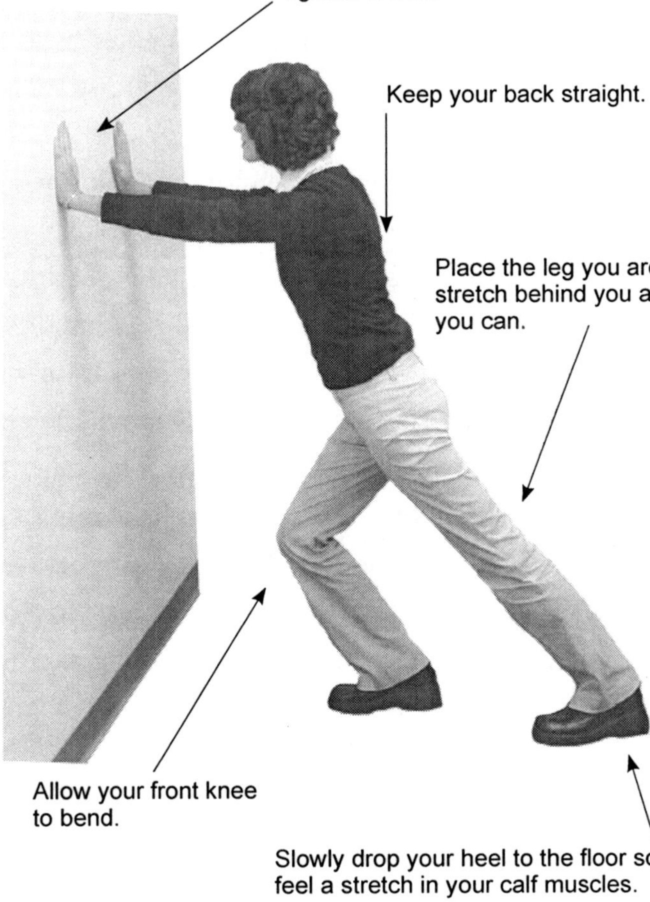

Desk Push-Ups

Desk Push-Ups are a great way to improve the strength of the pec major muscles. To do this exercise, start by placing both hands on the edge of your desk. Step back so that your body is angled about 45 degrees from the floor and hold your body away from your desk with your arms straight. Bend your elbows and lower your body all the way down until your chest touches the front edge of the desk, then straighten your arms again to raise your body back up. Repeat this exercise for a total of 10-20 repetitions.

If you haven't done much strength training, this exercise may seem very difficult or impossible at first. If you are unable to do at least ten push-ups where you touch your chest to your desk, start out by only going down halfway. It is important to do at least ten repetitions in order to work the muscle enough to increase strength. As you become stronger, you will be able to drop your body closer and closer to your desk. One other thing that you can do if you find this exercise too challenging at first is to place your feet closer to your desk. The closer your feet are to your desk, the easier this exercise will be, at least to a point. You can modify this exercise as you need as long as you are able to do the exercise comfortably.

Desk Push-Ups

Benefits: Pec Major Strength

Equipment Needed: Desk

Time / Repetitions: 10-20 Repetitions

Keep your back straight.

Place your feet back far enough so that your body makes a 45 degree angle to the floor.

Place your hands on the edge of your desk.

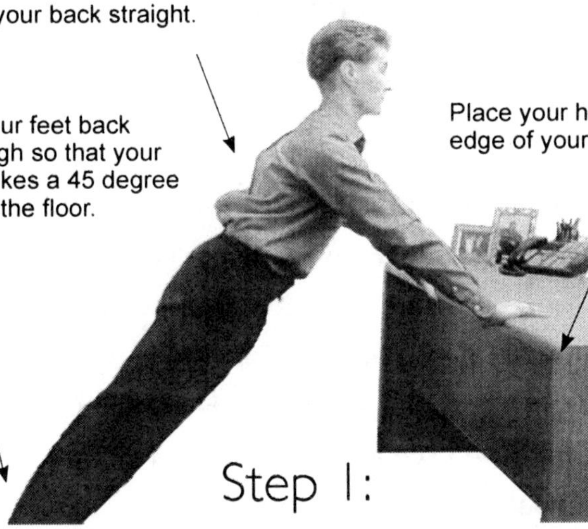

Step 1:

Bend your elbows and lower your chest to your desk, then push yourself back up.

Keep your back straight.

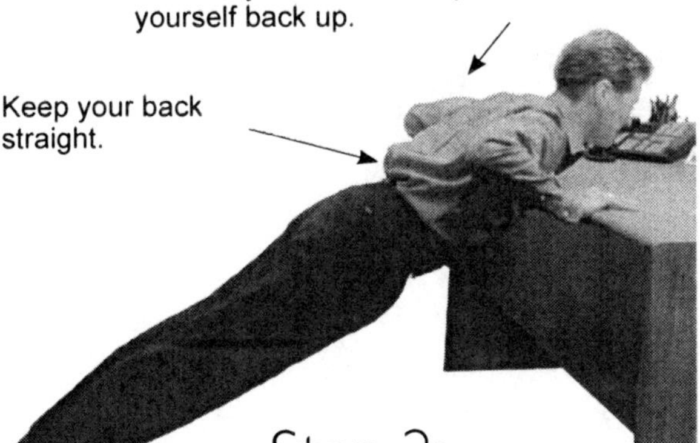

Step 2:

The Stick-Em Up Stretch

The Stick-Em Up Stretch is great for decreasing the tension of the pec minor muscle, allowing the shoulders to roll back to a healthier posture and decreasing any tingling and numbness in the arms that may be present. This stretch is called the Stick-Em Up stretch because you start by assuming the posture often seen in old Western movies when the villain says "Stick 'em up!" Your upper arms should be parallel to the floor, with your elbows bent 90 degrees so that your hands are raised above your head with your palms facing forward. With your arms in that position, step into a doorway so that your forearms rest against the door frame. Be sure that your feet are centered within the doorway. Gently push your hips forward until you feel a stretch in your upper chest and shoulders. Hold this position without bouncing for 30-45 seconds, then step away from the doorway and allow your hands to drop to your side.

It is important that this stretch be done on a daily basis. When the pec minor is tight, it causes one of the major components of the Foreward Head Posture—the dreaded forward shoulders and the resultant hunching of the upper back.

The Stick-Em Up Stretch

Benefits: Pec Minor Flexibility

Equipment Needed: Doorway

Time / Repetitions: 30-45 Seconds

Face your palms forward.

Bend your elbows 90 degrees and raise your upper arms so that they are parallel to the floor.

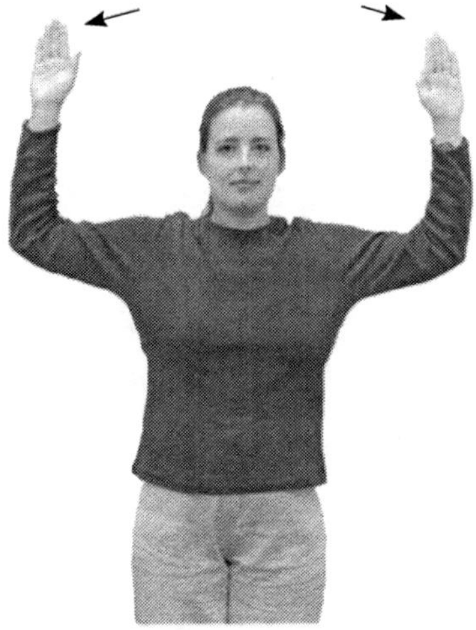

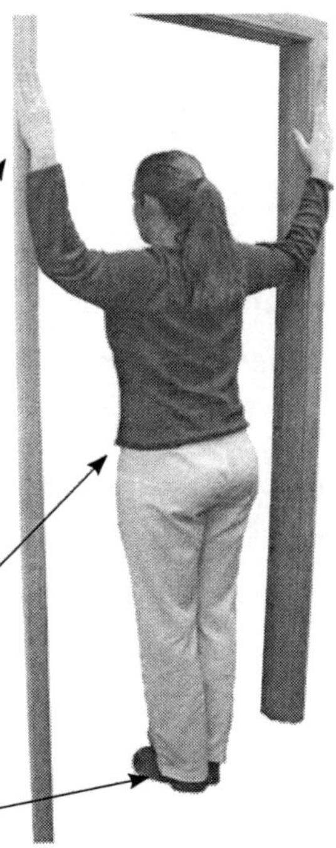

Place your forearms against a door frame.

Stand up straight and gently lean forward until you feel a stretch in your upper pecs. Hold this position for 30-45 seconds.

Bring your feet into the doorway so that you are not bending forward.

Dumbbell Curls

The Dumbbell Curl is the simplest, most effective way to improve the strength in the biceps muscle. To do this exercise, start by standing up straight and holding one dumbbell in each hand; palms facing forward. Using only the muscles in your arm, lift the weight up to your shoulder by bending your elbow. Once you raise the weight as far as you can, gently lower it back down again. One entire repetition should take three to four seconds.

It is important when doing this exercise to keep your elbows locked to your side and not move them forward or backward—that's cheating. The other important thing is to keep your body from swaying back when you raise the dumbbell—that's also cheating. My favorite way to do this exercise is to alternate hands so that while I am raising a dumbbell with one hand, I am lowering the dumbbell in the other. But you may prefer to only exercise one arm at a time. Either way is okay as long as you do 10-15 repetitions with each arm. As with the other exercises which utilize weights, if you are able to do 16 repetitions, you need to increase the weight you are lifting. If you are unable to do ten repetitions, you will need to decrease the weight you are using.

This exercise is particularly effective in reducing the tightness in your biceps if you immediately follow it up with the Biceps Door Stretch.

Dumbbell Curls

Benefits:	Biceps Strength
Equipment Needed:	Pair of Dumbbells
Time / Repetitions:	10-15 Repetitions for Each Arm

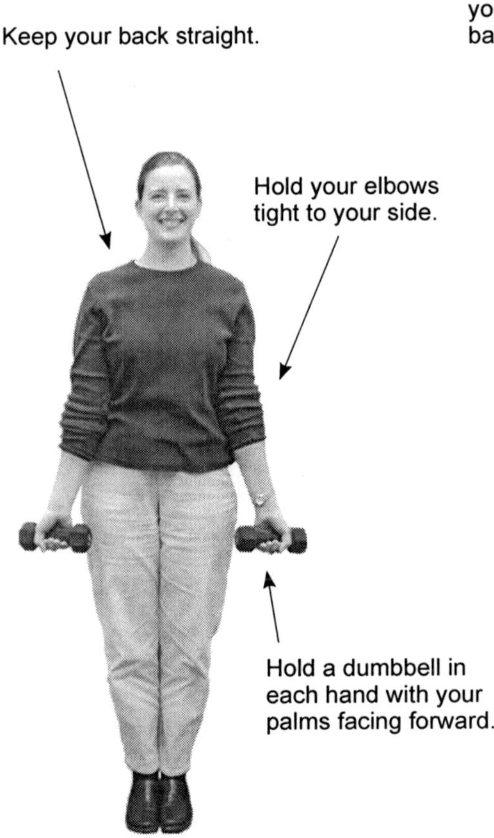

Step 1:

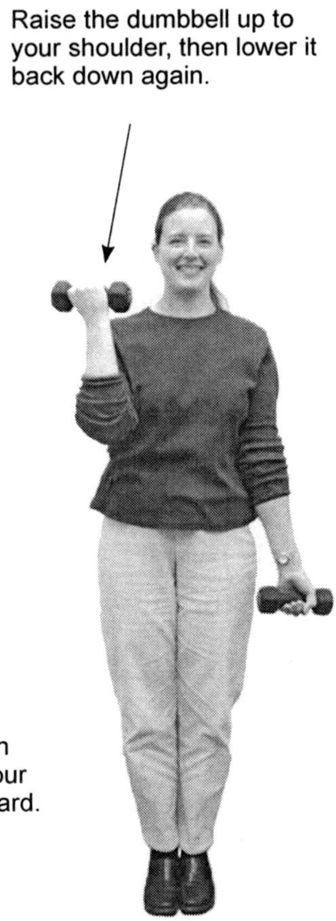
Raise the dumbbell up to your shoulder, then lower it back down again.

Step 2:

Chair Dips

This exercise does wonders for the strength of the triceps muscle and, to a lesser degree, the muscles in the front of the shoulder. To do this exercise, start by leaning against the edge of your chair, place your hands on either side and grip the arms of your chair. Move your hips about 12"-18" away from the edge of the chair by moving your feet forward, while keeping your arms straight and your hands gripping the arms of the chair. Keeping your back straight and your head up, lower your hips as far as you can toward the floor by bending your elbows, then straighten your arms to lift yourself up again. Repeat this exercise for a total of 10-15 repetitions.

Depending on your condition, you may find this exercise to be very difficult. Don't worry if you cannot do ten repetitions, or even five repetitions for that matter, when you first try this exercise. If you just keep doing Chair Dips, you will gradually become stronger and they will become easier.

One trick that works well when you cannot do ten repetitions of a particular exercise is to break up the routine into smaller chunks. You may want to do five repetitions, take a short break, then do five more. You can even break it into two-repetition chunks if you have to, and do two repetitions five times throughout the day.

Chair Dips

Benefits:	Triceps Strength
Equipment Needed:	Chair
Time / Repetitions:	10-15 Repetitions

Step 1:

Look straight ahead.

Place your feet out in front of you far enough so that there is 12"-18" of space between your hips and the chair seat.

Place your hands either on the arm rests or the seat of a stable chair.

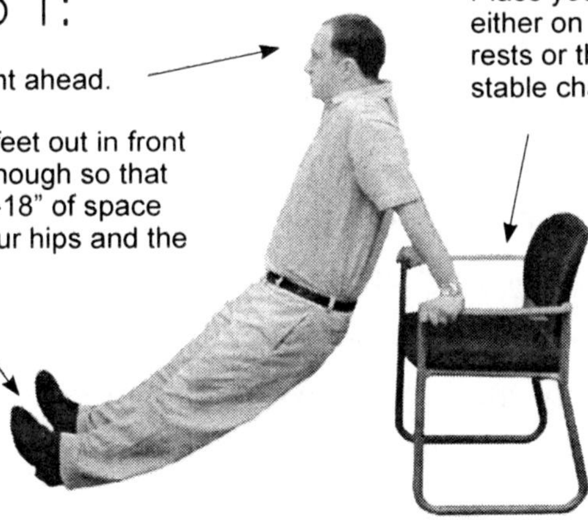

Step 2:

Look straight ahead.

Keep your legs straight.

Lower your hips toward the floor by bending your elbows, then push yourself back up again.

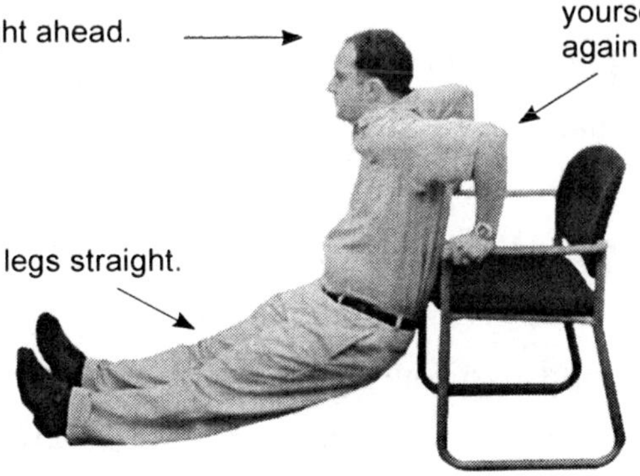

The Overhead Press

The Overhead Press is a great overall exercise to improve the strength in the triceps and shoulders. Begin by grasping a pair of dumbbells and raising them up to your shoulders, palms facing forward as shown in the picture on the opposite page. Raise the weights above your head by straightening your arms and bring the weights together so that they touch. Then gently lower the weights back down to the level of your shoulders. Repeat for a total of 10-15 repetitions.

If you have never done this exercise before, your arms may feel fairly wobbly and uncoordinated. This is normal and will go away after a couple of weeks of doing the exercise. It is also common for people who have not done this exercise before to feel like their muscles are not getting a very good workout. This happens because you are asking your muscles to work in a way that they are not used to, so they will be a bit uncoordinated. Just keep doing the exercise and you will eventually feel your muscles begin to get a good workout.

It is important when doing the Overhead Press that two basic safety rules are followed. The first is that you should not use a weight that is too heavy for you. If you cannot do ten repetitions, you need to use a lighter weight. The second is that you should not use dumbbells that have removable plates. Instead, use solid-cast, one-piece dumbbells that cannot come apart and cause injury when they are raised above your head.

The Overhead Press

Benefits:	Shoulder and Triceps Strength
Equipment Needed:	Pair of Dumbbells
Time / Repetitions:	10-15 Repetitions

Hold a dumbbell in each hand with your palms facing forward.

Sit up straight.

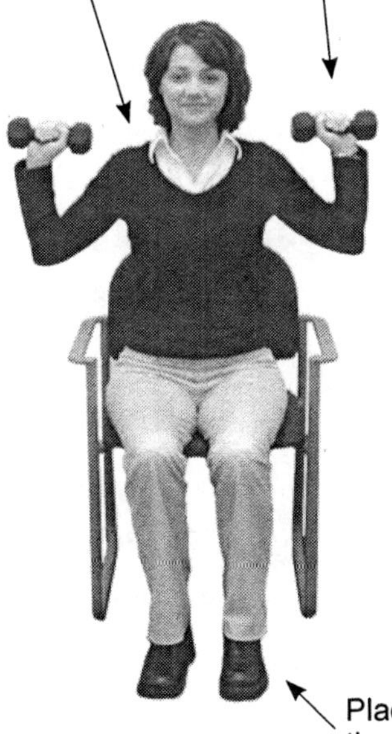

Place your feet flat on the floor.

Step 1:

Raise the dumbbells above your head as high as you can until they gently touch.

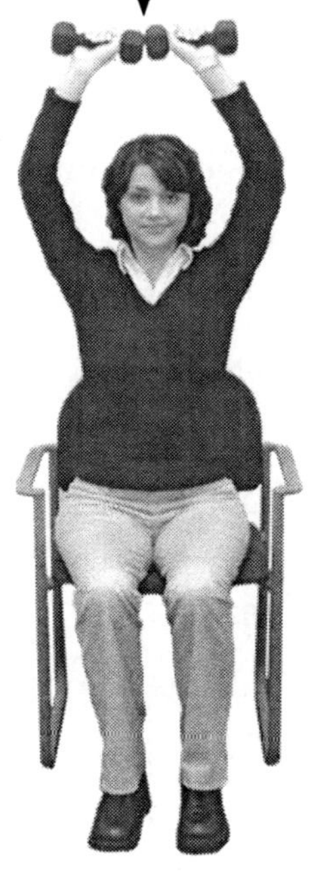

Step 2:

The Biceps Door Stretch

The Biceps Door Stretch is a very effective way to decrease the tightness in the biceps muscles. To do this stretch, begin by gripping the frame of a door so that your thumb points toward the floor as shown in the picture on the opposite page. Slide your hand up to just below the level of your shoulder. Turn your body so that your arm is directly behind you and your shoulders are parallel to the wall. Gently push your pelvis forward until you feel a stretch in your upper arm. Hold the stretch for 30-45 seconds, then switch arms and do the same. When you switch arms, you will have to move to the other side of the door frame.

This stretch can be a bit tricky. If you do not feel a stretch in your arm, you are probably doing one of two things incorrectly. The first and most common mistake that most people make is that their shoulders are not parallel to the wall where the door is located. Make sure that your shoulders are lined up with the wall and not in a straight line with your arm. The second mistake is not raising your hand high enough behind you. This is easily corrected by simply sliding your hand up further. As long as your shoulders are square with the wall, you will eventually reach a point where you feel a stretch in your biceps muscle.

You can make this stretch even more effective by performing it immediately following your Dumbbell Curls when your muscles are nice and warm.

The Biceps Door Stretch

Benefits:	Biceps Flexibility
Equipment Needed:	Doorway
Time / Repetitions:	30-45 Seconds on Each Side

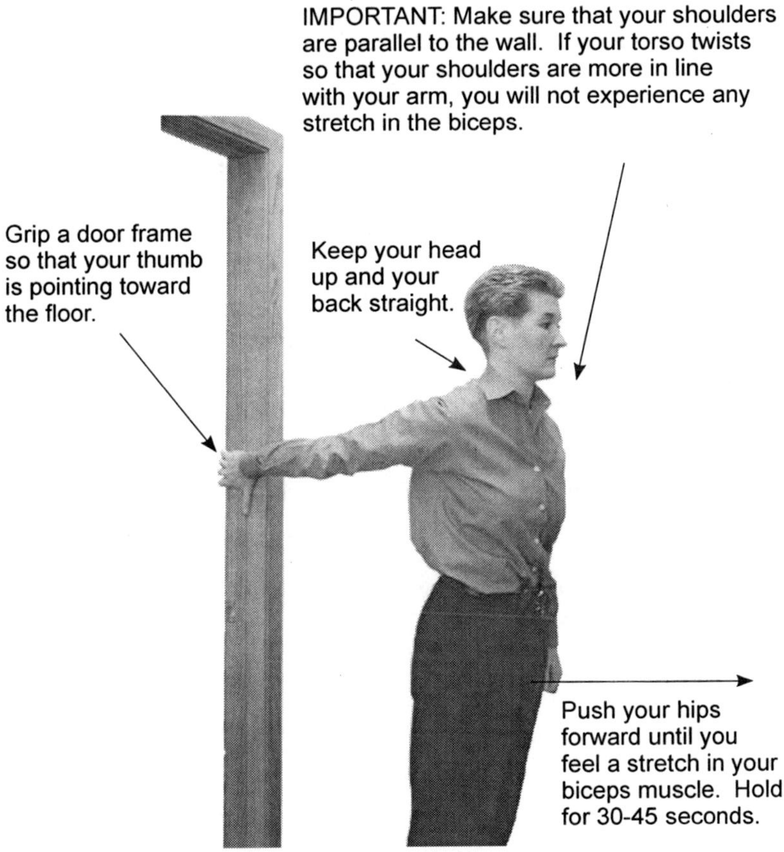

The Wrist Stretch

The Wrist Stretch is designed to decrease the tension in your forearms and wrists. To do this stretch straighten out one of your arms and allow your wrist to relax. Take your other hand and gently pull your wrist into further flexion as shown in Step 1 in the picture on the opposite page. Hold this stretch for 30-45 seconds, then switch directions and pull your hand upwards to stretch the forearm flexors. Hold this stretch for 30-45 seconds, then switch hands.

To get the most out of this stretch, it is best to do it at least twice per day; three times would be even better. Be careful not to pull too hard on your hand and over-stretch the muscles in your forearms. Those muscles are fairly small and can be strained easily.

If you suffer from Carpal Tunnel Syndrome, this stretch may cause some tingling in your hands. Minor tingling is probably not a major concern and should improve after a few days of doing this stretch. However, if the pain or tingling in your hands is moderate to severe, only do the Wrist Stretch to the point where the pain begins, then back off a bit.

When you experience tingling in your hands by doing the Wrist Stretch, it indicates that the median nerve which runs through the center of your wrist is being pinched. You don't want to pinch it too much or you may cause the nerve to become irritated or injured. So remember, a little tingling is okay when doing the Wrist Stretch, but a lot of tingling or pain is a sign that you are overdoing it a bit.

The Wrist Stretch

Benefits:	Wrist and Forearm Flexibility
Equipment Needed:	None
Time / Repetitions:	30-45 Seconds

Step 1:

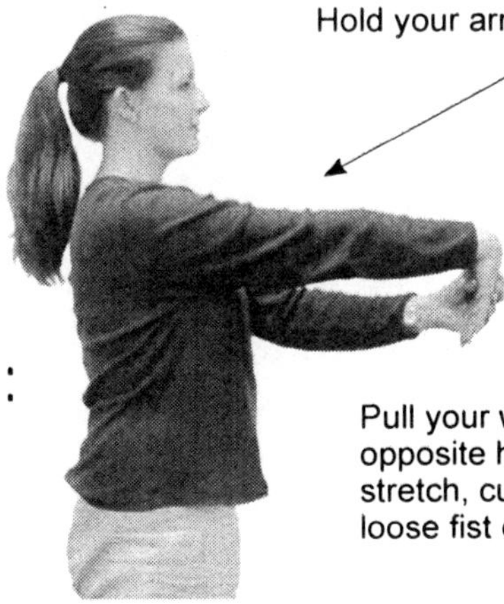

Hold your arm out straight.

Pull your wrist forward with your opposite hand. For more of a stretch, curl your fingers into a loose fist during this stretch.

Step 2:

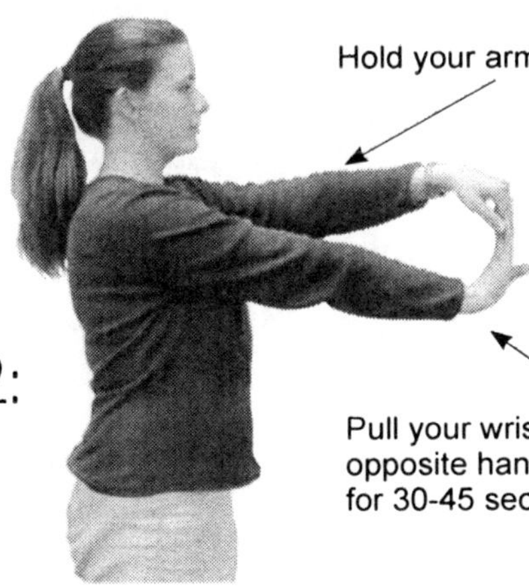

Hold your arm out straight.

Pull your wrist back with your opposite hand. Hold this stretch for 30-45 seconds.

10

Vital Step Five: Eliminate Toxins

After 16 years of practice, the single most beneficial program in my office other than chiropractic adjustments is liver detoxification. I have assisted thousands of patients and have seen dramatic changes in people's health, diet, and overall wellbeing.

A feeling of being in charge of your health comes to people that complete a detox program mostly because the results are so dramatic and it is seen that what you eat can have a huge affect on overall health and wellness. Following a detox, people report an overall improvement in their energy level, less dependence on caffeine and sugar for energy, and less mood swings. I am going to explain in detail the why of detox and give some assistance in ways to eliminate the toxins in your life.

The first thing to understand is that the liver is the main organ of detoxification. Although the focus of detox is on the liver, every other system in the body is compromised if your liver is not functioning properly. That's because many of the toxins to which we are exposed are fat soluble, meaning they cannot be directly excreted in the water-based urine, but instead are attracted to fatty cell membranes in our bodies. This attraction allows them to be easily transported inside of the cells where they can sequester and exert their toxic effects. These toxins become permanent residents of our systems, challenging our entire body function, including liver, kidney, heart, brain, colon, lungs, skin, and hormonal systems. Toxic overload is the major contributor to a hyperactive or hypoactive immune system.

It should be obvious that with fewer toxins to contend with, you will experience more energy, more vitality and be in better health. The challenge then is to find a detoxification program designed to change these fat-soluble toxins into a water-soluble form so they can then be easily flushed from the system through the kidneys or colon. First let's see what these toxins are and where they come from.

What are Toxins?

According to the Environmental Protection Agency (EPA), over 4 billion pounds of toxic chemicals are released by industry into the nation's environment each year, including 72 million pounds of recognized carcinogens. Currently, there are only 650 substances whose release into the environment is tracked by the EPA - which represents less than 1% of the over 75,000 chemicals manufactured in the U.S. To make matters worse, the EPA has never systematically reviewed the available environmental health data to ascertain just how toxic the vast majority of these environmental contaminants are.

Even if you live in a part of the country where you can avoid most of the industrial contaminants that are present in the big cities, it is almost impossible to avoid them. Why? Because toxic chemicals are everywhere! They are in amalgam dental fillings, fluoridated and chlorinated water, present as additives in our food and personal care products, in the air we breathe and the water we drink. In today's world, we live in a sea of toxins.

It is true that laws are being passed on a regular basis in an effort to protect the environment from these toxins. However, environmental protection laws are usually not passed until toxic levels of chemicals have already created a great deal of harm to the environment; not to mention the fact that new chemicals are being introduced into the marketplace so quickly, that adequate safety testing and regulation rarely happen. Likewise, science continues to discover new health threats from existing chemicals, such as endocrine system impairments from estrogen-mimicking pesticides.

Since 1976, the EPA has been conducting the National Human Adipose Tissue Survey (NHATS). NHATS is an annual program that collects and chemically analyzes a nationwide sample of fat tissue samples from a variety of animals for the presence of toxic compounds. The objective of the program is to detect and quantify the prevalence of toxic compounds in the general population.

In 1982 the EPA expanded beyond their normal list to look for the presence of 54 different environmental chemical toxins. Their results were astounding. Five of these chemicals—dioxin, styrene, dichlorobenzene, xylene, and ethylphenol—were found in 100 percent of the tissues they sampled. Another nine chemicals were found in over 90 percent of all samples.

Additional studies yielded similar results. A study of four-year-old children in Michigan revealed the presence of DDT in 70 percent, PCB in 50 percent, and PBB in 21 percent. Breast feeding was the primary source of exposure for these individuals. These ongoing assessments have shown quite clearly it is not a question of if we are carrying a burden of toxic compounds, it is a question of how much and how they affect our health.

How Do Toxins Get Into Your Body?

In your day-to-day life, you are exposed to toxins on numerous levels, some within your control, such as the foods you consume, and some totally outside your control. Accordingly, it makes sense to learn something about the various kinds of exposure that you encounter daily in order to make informed choices to reduce your overall level of toxic intake.

How Do These Toxins Affect Your Health?

The 20th century, with its promise of "Better Living through Chemistry," brought a host of chemical toxin-related illnesses, often referred to as environmental illness. Recent articles in the medical literature have shown the rate of cancers not associated with smoking are higher for those born after 1940 than before, and that this increase in cancer rate is due to environmental factors other than smoking. New medical diagnoses include sick (closed) building syndrome, and multiple chemical sensitivity (MCS), both of which are known to be related to overexposure to environmental contaminants. The primary action of the major pesticide classes and solvents is to disrupt neurological function. In addition to being neurotoxic, these compounds are profoundly toxic to the immune and endocrine systems. The adverse health effects are not limited only to those systems, as these compounds can cause a variety of dermatological, gastrointestinal, genitourinary, respiratory, musculoskeletal, and cardiological problems as well.

Adverse Immune Effects

Environmental chemicals have a wide range of effects on immune system function, ranging from decreased cell-mediated immunity (with a decrease in ability to fight infections and tumors) to increased sensitivity (allergy) and autoimmunity.

Chemically-exposed individuals often present with elevated antibodies to certain body tissues, which means their body is attacking itself. Another word for these conditions are 'autoimmune disorders,' which are at epidemic proportions in our country.

Toxin-Associated Cancers

Several hundred of the 75,000 chemicals currently being released into the environment are known or suspected carcinogens (cancer causing). These chemicals interfere with the normal cell growth and development, resulting in areas of tissue that grow out of control. The more toxic exposure an individual has, the greater risk they have of developing a cancer.

When looking at the correlation between toxic chemical exposure and the rate of cancer, a strong association becomes obvious. Men born in the 1940s had twice the cancer incidence as those born from 1888-1897, even when smoking was factored out. Women born in the 1940s had 50 percent more total cancers, with 30 percent more cancer not linked to smoking in Caucasian women. Cancers in children are at an all-time high, especially brain cancers in those who have been exposed to pesticides. Several studies have also shown that leukemias and myelomas are associated exposures to environmental toxins, especially industrial solvents.

Because many of the carcinogenic toxins resemble hormones in the body – especially estrogen – cancers tend to form in tissues that are sensitive to these hormones; hence the dramatic increase in breast cancer, testicular cancer and ovarian cancer.

Neurotoxicity

Neurotoxicity simply means that a particular compound is toxic to the nervous system. Most of the major classes of pesticides are neurotoxins by design – they kill pests by attacking their nervous system. Numerous studies have shown that exposure to pesticides and agricultural fertilizers contribute to the development of Alzheimer's disease, Parkinson's disease and Multiple Sclerosis (MS), as well as neuropathies in the hands and feet.

Even more disturbing is that some of the compounds that have been shown to be neurotoxic in the laboratory are actually used as food additives, such as the flavor-enhancer monosodium glutamate (MSG) and Aspartame (NutraSweet®). Each of these compounds is referred to as an 'excitoneurotoxin', meaning that its toxic effects are from over-stimulating the nerves. Conditions like attention deficit disorder, convulsions, obesity and learning disorders have all been linked to consumption of chemical flavoring agents in the laboratory.

Endocrine Toxicity

In addition to the well-documented estrogenic effects of certain toxins, actual damage to the endocrine organs can also occur. The most common symptoms of toxic damage to the endocrine system are:

- *Sleep disturbances or changes in energy level or mood.*
- *Alterations in weight, appetite and bowel function.*
- *Change in sexual interest and function, menstrual change.*
- *Changes in temperature perception, sweating, or flushing.*
- *Alteration of hair growth and skin texture.*
- *Disruption of normal thyroid function; and Infertility in men.*
- *With the exception of reproductive effects, most of these endocrine symptoms occur only after immunological and/or neurological symptoms are already present.*

Removing the Toxic Overload in our Bodies

Juice Detoxing

According to Dr. Sandra Cabot, physician and nutrition author, raw fruit and vegetable juices help to cleanse and re-energize your liver. The pectin in apple juice helps to remove excess cholesterol and heavy metals from the digestive tract, reducing the workload of the liver. Try a simple three-day detox by drinking a glass of freshly juiced apple and beet juice before every meal. Also try drinking a glass of water with one to three teaspoons of fresh lemon juice every morning before breakfast. This helps to flush and clear the liver.

Detox Foods

Foods rich in antioxidants help to stimulate and cleanse the liver and remove toxins from the body. I recommend adding high antioxidant foods such as beets, eggplant, carrots, red onion, artichokes, grapefruit and grapes to your diet. Other foods that promote liver health include cruciferous vegetables, onions and the spice turmeric. Also add more ginger, which increases blood circulation for better removal of toxins, and garlic, which is rich in the mineral selenium for liver health. According to a study published in "Digestive Diseases and Sciences," people with a selenium deficiency have greater risks of liver problems and disease.

Daily Detox

Regular detoxing helps to keep the liver healthy and decongested. Daily ways to improve liver health recommended by Dr. Cabot include drinking plenty of water and getting fresh air, as well as regular exercise that makes you sweat a little. She also suggests adding a cup of bath salts to a warm water bath to help draw out toxins as you soak.

Sweat

Sweating removes harmful chemicals through your skin and makes a great way to detox naturally. You can start simply by exercising more often. Focus on aerobics-based exercise such as running and cycling. These activities encourage blood circulation rather than building muscle mass. Saunas and spas are another way to sweat. You can also take a detox bath using hot water mixed with 1 cup of Epsom salts or baking soda. That helps open up the pores and leach harmful chemicals out of your skin. You may want to dry brush your skin before you bathe, which removes dead cells and helps clear the pores.

Medically Supervised Cleansing Programs

In my office, I oversee a multitude of cleansing programs to free the body of these toxic substances. I use mostly the Metagenics programs and line of supplements to assist in detoxification. The detoxification programs designed by Metagenics help reduce the amount of toxins we ingest and assist the body's natural processes for eliminating toxins already in your system. These programs can focus on the liver, the intestine, metal detox, and even address pH balance in the body. Please refer to youcanbewell.com for detailed information about the program and how it can help you.

Tips for Avoiding Toxins

It's impossible to avoid all environmental toxins, but you can limit your exposure by following a few tips:

- *As much as possible, eat organic produce and free-range, organic foods.*
- *Rather than eating fish, which is largely contaminated with PCBs and mercury, consume a high-quality purified fish or cod liver oil.*
- *Avoid processed foods - remember that they're processed with chemicals!*
- *Only use natural cleaning products in your home*
- *Switch over to natural brands of toiletries*
- *Remove any metal fillings as they're a major source of mercury. Be sure to have this done by a qualified biological dentist.*
- *Avoid using artificial air fresheners, dryer sheets, fabric softeners or other synthetic fragrances as they can pollute the air you are breathing.*
- *Avoid artificial food additives of all kind, including artificial sweeteners and MSG*
- *Get plenty of safe sun exposure to boost your vitamin D levels and your immune system (you'll be better able to fight disease).*
- *Have your tap water tested and, if contaminants are found, install an appropriate water filter on all your faucets (even those in your shower or bath).*

11

Wellness Lifestyle Tips

Regular chiropractic care, eating a healthy diet, taking vitamin supplements, keeping your weight under control and stress management are all part of an overall wellness lifestyle that, if followed, results in a longer, healthier and pain-free life. Here is a list of basic tips to help you maintain a healthier, more vibrant body.

Regular Chiropractic Care

The chiropractic approach to healthcare is holistic, meaning that it addresses your overall health. Numerous studies have demonstrated that chiropractic care is one of the most effective treatments for back pain, neck pain, headaches, whiplash, sports injuries and many other types of musculoskeletal problems. It has even been shown to be effective in reducing high blood pressure, decreasing the frequency of childhood ear infections (otitis media) and improving the symptoms of asthma.

Chiropractic is so much more than simply a means of relieving pain. Ultimately, the goal of the chiropractic treatment is to restore the body to its natural state of optimal health. In order to accomplish this, chiropractors use a variety of treatment methods, including manual adjustments, massage, trigger point therapy, nutrition, exercise rehabilitation, and massage, as well as counseling on lifestyle issues that impact your health. Since the body has a remarkable ability to heal itself and to maintain its own health, my primary focus is simply to remove those things which interfere with the body's normal healing ability.

Chiropractors understand that within each of us is an innate wisdom, a health energy, which will express itself as perfect health and well-being if we simply allow it to. Therefore, the focus of chiropractic care is simply to remove any physiological blocks to the proper expression of the body's innate wisdom. Once these subluxations are removed, health is the natural consequence.

Just like continuing an exercise program and eating well in order to sustain the benefits of exercise and proper diet, it is necessary to continue chiropractic care to ensure the health of your musculoskeletal system. When you make routine chiropractic care a part of your lifestyle, you avoid many of the aches and pains that so many people suffer through, your joints will last longer and you will be able to engage in more of the activities you love.

Many years ago, dentists convinced everyone that the best time to go to the dentist is before your teeth hurt – that routine dental care will help your teeth remain healthy for a long time. It is important to remember that, just like your teeth, your spine experiences normal wear and tear – you walk, drive, sit, lift, sleep and bend. Regular chiropractic care can help you feel better, move with more freedom, and stay healthier throughout your lifetime. Although you can enjoy the benefits of chiropractic care even if you are only treated for a short time, the real benefits come into play when you make chiropractic care a part of your lifestyle.

Maintain a Healthy Body Weight

Most people know that excessive body weight contributes to the development of a number of conditions, such as coronary heart disease, diabetes, high blood pressure, and colon cancer. However, it may also be a major contributing factor for the development of low back pain. The spine is designed to carry a certain amount of body weight. When it is exposed to the excess pressure of being overweight, the spine becomes stressed and, over time, can suffer structural damage. Being overweight significantly contributes to symptoms associated with osteoporosis, osteoarthritis (OA), rheumatoid arthritis (RA), degenerative disc disease (DDD), spinal stenosis, and spondylolisthesis.

In addition to back pain, those who are overweight may suffer from fatigue, as well as difficulty breathing and shortness of breath during short periods of exercise. If the fatigue and shortness of breath causes one to avoid activity and exercise, then this can indirectly lead to back pain as lack of exercise contributes to many common forms of back pain.

If you are currently overweight and suffer from low back pain, talk to your doctor of chiropractic about effective ways to lose weight. Not only will your back pain improve, but you will decrease your risk of most major degenerative diseases at the same time.

Sleep on a Good Mattress

Good health and sleep are closely linked. Just as we improve our eating habits for better health, we should also improve our sleep habits. Sleep deprivation is a costly problem in our society, both fiscally and physically. Sleep should be a priority and not just a negotiable need determined by our busy schedules. Good sleep not only reduces costly back problems but also helps to prepare us for a more productive, alert and safe day ahead. Here are some tips to help you select the proper mattress for you:

- *Personal preference should ultimately determine what mattress to purchase. Any mattress that helps someone sleep without pain and stiffness is the best mattress for that individual. There is no single mattress that works for all people with low back pain.*

- *Find a mattress with sufficient back support to reduce low back pain. A good mattress should provide support while allowing for the natural curves and alignment of the spine. Medium-firm mattresses usually provide more back pain relief than firm mattresses.*
- *Know when it's time to get a new mattress. If an old mattress sags visibly in the middle, it is probably time to purchase a new one. Putting boards under a sagging mattress is only a short-term fix and may cause more back problems and low back pain in the long run.*
- *Be wary of mattress advertising gimmicks. Claims that a mattress is "orthopedic" or "medically-approved" should be viewed skeptically. There has not been extensive medical research or controlled clinical trials on the topic of mattresses and low back pain. You must determine whether or not extra features on a mattress make it more comfortable or supportive for your back.*

In our clinic we recommend Pro-Adjuster Sleep System by iSleep. The leading contributing factor to sleeping difficulties is the actual sleeping surface. This mattress system includes pressure relieving foam, dual air chambers, and patented inner coil design. A testimonial to the quality and the certainty of the ProAdjuster Sleep System by iSleep is that each and every system that is ordered comes with an unconditional 30 Day "Test Rest" program. This unmatched policy means that if for any reason our patients are not completely satisfied with the Sleep

System for 30 full nights, they can return it – with absolutely no obligation. Mention Dr. Maj and get a custom fitting.

Wear Orthotics

Your feet are your foundation! In our clinic, we start all examinations from the feet up. You cannot expect your million dollar house to stand if it is on a faulty foundation. The same holds true for your body. Orthotics are custom fitted inserts that you place into your shoes to keep your feet functioning correctly. They support you when you stand, walk, or run. And they help protect your spine, bones, and soft tissues from damaging stress as you move around. Your feet perform better when all their muscles, arches, and bones are in their ideal stable positions.

The foot is constructed with three arches which, when properly maintained, give exceptional supportive strength. These three arches form a supporting vault that distributes the weight of the entire body. If there is compromise of one arch in the foot, the other arches must compensate and are subject to additional stresses, which usually leads to further compromise.

By stabilizing and balancing your feet, orthotics enhance your body's performance and efficiency, reduce pain, and contribute to your total body wellness. Since the average person spends almost two-thirds of their day in shoes, it's important to make sure that they provide optimal support.

The most popular brand of orthotics (and the brand I use in my clinic) is Foot Levelers. Foot Levelers orthotics support all three arches in your feet, thereby creating a stable foundation upon which to build proper body posture. Their support is minimally invasive meaning that the arches are supported yet the strength of the intrinsic muscles of the foot is maintained. The hard, plastic orthotics cause the muscles to atrophy and are very uncomfortable to the user.

Drink More Water

Water is the most abundant nutrient in the body, accounting for around 60–65 percent of your total weight. It is also the least forgiving of all the nutrients you consume. You can survive for weeks without food, but for only a couple of days without water. Water is responsible for the transport of nutrients, oxygen and waste products, as well as regulating your body temperature and serving as the medium in which all of your body's chemical reactions take place. Most people do not drink enough pure clean water.

Drinking an adequate amount of clean water every day is one of the most overlooked, but simplest ways of keeping your body healthy. Water is used to help the body cleanse itself of toxins and metabolic waste. Although drinking water has become more popular over the past several years, many people still do not consume enough water. Instead, they drink coffee, tea, juices and soft drinks and figure that they get enough fluids. It is true that when you drink these things you are consuming water. However, along with the water, you are also consuming a lot of other ingredients that the body will need to ultimately eliminate, so the potential beneficial effect of the water is somewhat negated. To make matters worse, drinks that contain caffeine, such as coffee, tea and soft drinks, actually cause more water loss than the amount of water they contain, resulting in a net loss of water.

Ideally, the average person should consume around ten cups of water per day, or just over a half gallon. Some of this water is found in the food and beverages you consume, so you don't have to drink an entire half-gallon of water every day. An easy way to accomplish this is to buy a 1.5 liter bottle of water from the local grocery store and to drink that amount of water every day. If you exercise heavily, you may have to drink two of those 1.5 liter bottles of water each day. By drinking enough water, you will be helping your body to remain healthy. It is by far the cheapest health insurance you can buy.

Eat More Fruits and Vegetables

People know that they should eat more fruit and vegetables in their diet, but most people don't do it. It seems lately that the four major food groups of the American diet have gone from dairy, fruits and vegetables, grains, and meat to sugar, fat, salt and caffeine. Because of the easy availability of fast foods and snack foods, we have lost our taste for fruits and vegetables; especially vegetables. It is not uncommon for many people to go for weeks without consuming a single serving of fresh vegetables. This is not good.

The human body evolved with a diet high in fruits and vegetables, and is dependent on many of the compounds unique to plant foods in order to operate correctly. If you don't consume enough of these plant compounds, your energy level will suffer along with your overall health. Most people are shocked at how much better they feel when they cut down on the fast foods and snack foods and increase their fruit and vegetable intake.

If you find it difficult to work in several servings of fruits and vegetables into your routine every day, you may find it helpful to supplement your diet with what is called a "greens" supplement, which is a highly concentrated powder of fruits, vegetables and antioxidants.

Increasing your consumption of fruits and vegetables is an important way to improve your overall health. The key is to make it part of your lifestyle - to make it a new habit.

Cut Down on Sugar

In a recent study done by the USDA, it was reported that the average American consumes 134 pounds of refined sugar every year, or approximately 20 teaspoons of sugar per day. As hard as this may be to believe, consider the following facts:

- *A 12 oz. can of PepsiTM contains 10 teaspoons of sugar*
- *A 2 oz. package of candy contains 11 teaspoons of sugar*
- *A 16 oz. cup of lemonade contains 13 teaspoons of sugar*
- *A cup of Frosted FlakesTM contains 4 teaspoons of sugar*

This high level of sugar intake is very unhealthy and contributes to obesity, Type II diabetes, heart disease (due to elevated triglycerides), kidney stones, dental cavities, chronic tiredness and reactive hypoglycemia. Decreasing your sugar intake is as simple as avoiding foods which are high in refined sugars, such as soft drinks, candy, cake and donuts, as well as most condiments. When you purchase sweetened food, look for products that are sweetened with apple juice or stevia, rather than sugar or high-fructose corn syrup.

Get Into the Light

One of the most important nutrients for your mind and body speeds toward you at 186,000 miles per second from more than 93 million miles away. This nutrient is called sunlight. Most people don't think of sunlight as a nutrient, but it is. Sunlight is necessary for regulating proper hormone function, calcium absorption, bone health as well as a normal daily sleep-wake cycle (circadian rhythm). In fact, if you don't get enough sunlight in your daily 'light diet,' you can suffer deficiency symptoms, such as:

- *Seasonal depression (Seasonal Affective Disorder)*
- *Poor quality of sleep*
- *Loss in work performance (especially in night-shift workers)*
- *Disrupted melatonin regulation*
- *Depressed cortical brain activity*
- *Depressed immune function*

Unfortunately, the light to which most of us are exposed each day comes from manmade sources, such as fluorescent, sodium and incandescent lights that do not produce full-spectrum sunlight. Numerous studies have shown that these limited-spectrum artificial light sources can make students irritable in school, reduce production among factory workers and make office workers sluggish. In one study, researchers even found that calcium absorption dropped off in the elderly who spent their days indoors during the winter, while those who spent time under full-spectrum lighting had an increase in calcium absorption.

Getting enough full-spectrum light can give your mood a tremendous boost. Light can help reduce stress, help you feel happier and improve your ability to concentrate. To make sure that you are getting enough light in your diet, doctors recommend the following tips:

- *Try to spend at least 15 minutes outside every day; even when it's very cloudy. The full-spectrum daylight is still beneficial to your health.*
- *Begin using a light box during the fall and winter seasons, especially if you tend to get the winter blues.*
- *Stop wearing sunglasses as they create very unnatural light for your eyes. Sunglasses should only be worn when you need to protect your eyes from physical harm or very bright light.*

Take a Multivitamin

Many people don't think that they need to take vitamin supplements because, after all, the human body did not evolve to need supplements and as long as you eat a balanced diet, you can get everything that your body needs, right? While it is certainly true that people living a thousand years ago did not have multivitamins, they also did not have thousands of tons of toxic chemicals being pumped into their environment every year; they were not exposed to a constant man-made electromagnetic field from power lines and cell phones; they did not eat highly processed foods that contained artificial colors, flavors and preservatives; they were not sedentary; and they were not under constant stress at work and at home. Our bodies were simply not designed for a fast-paced, high-stress, highly processed lifestyle.

The reality is that we need to give our body some help in order to stay healthy in the world today. That's where supplements come in. Supplements help to ensure that your body gets all of the extra vitamins, minerals, antioxidants, fish oils, phytonutrients and probiotics necessary to function the way it should. You can find more information about the importance of vitamins on our website *www.YouCanBeWell.net*.

Keep Your Heart Healthy

Heart disease is currently the number one killer of adults in the United States. This is unfortunate because most heart disease is caused by poor lifestyle choices. The four big lifestyle changes you can make to ensure to maximize the health of your heart are exercise, maintaining a healthy body weight, taking a high quality vitamin supplement and stopping smoking.

Just as exercise is important to the health of your neuro-musculoskeletal system, it is also critical to the health of your heart. When you regularly exercise, your body becomes much more efficient at using oxygen and burning calories and your blood pressure is normalized. This decreases the stress on your heart. Another easy way to reduce the stress on your heart is to decrease the amount of body fat you carry around. It takes approximately one mile of additional blood vessels to supply one pound of additional fat. If you are twenty, thirty or fifty pounds overweight, it is easy to see how that extra body fat can place an undue burden on your heart.

Vitamins E and C and folic acid are the three most important nutritional supplements to take for your heart. Vitamin E is a powerful fat-soluble antioxidant which helps to prevent the cholesterol in your blood from becoming oxidized. High cholesterol levels in the blood, per se, are not that big of a deal. Cholesterol only becomes dangerous when it interacts with an oxidizing radical. Vitamin E helps to prevent this.

Vitamin C is important to help strengthen the walls of the arteries and prevent the development of cholesterol plaques inside the coronary arteries. Did you know that the arteries that are the most likely to develop cholesterol deposits are the ones that are close to the heart? The reason is that when the heart contracts, it pushes blood out with a great degree of force. If the walls of the arteries which are closest to the heart are not as strong as they should be, they will tend to momentarily stretch out like a balloon and cause small tears to the inside arterial wall as the rush of blood from the heart passes by. These small tears serve as a place where platelets and cholesterol form deposits. High levels of vitamin C reduce the number of tears in the arteries by strengthening the collagen tissues around the arteries, keeping them from expanding too much as blood pulses through.

The third vitamin which is important is one of the B-vitamins called folic acid. Folic acid, also called folacin, is important for reducing the level of homocysteine in the blood. Homocysteine is a metabolic by-product which can contribute significantly to the development of heart disease.

So, when you take your multivitamin while you are on your way to do your exercises, make sure that it contains at least 400 IU of vitamin E, at least 500 mg of vitamin C (1000 is even better) and 40 mcg of folic acid.

Stop Smoking

If you are a smoker, you are sick of hearing this, but.... it is REALLY important that you stop smoking! Smoking throughout the day is akin to living inside a burning building. Smoking degrades the collagen of your skin, causing premature wrinkling, destroys the cells inside your lungs, promotes heart disease, cataracts and cancer because of the oxidizing radicals released into the blood stream. It can also contribute to back pain by dehydrating the spinal discs.

Bone is a living tissue dependent on the functions and support provided by the other body systems. When these systems are not able to perform normally, bone is unable to rebuild itself. The formation of bone is particularly influenced by physical exercise and hormonal activity, both of which are adversely affected by cigarette smoking.

Smoking reduces the amount of oxygen in the blood and increases the level of harmful substances, such as carbon monoxide. In addition, nicotine causes a constriction of the small blood vessels that feed your spinal discs, shutting down their nutrient supply. Over time, the loss of normal blood supply leads to your discs becoming dehydrated and they begin to degenerate. Smoking is also known to cause an increase in estrogen loss in women who are perimenopausal or postmenopausal, which can result in a loss of bone density and increase your risk of developing osteoporosis.

There is no question that it is difficult to quit smoking. Many people who have quit say that it was the hardest thing they have ever done. But it is not impossible. People do it all the time. If you currently smoke and want to quit, there are a number of effective medical programs that can help you. Some people have also found complimentary therapies, such as acupuncture, to be helpful in quitting smoking.

How to Change Unhealthy Habits

There are three things that have to happen to successfully change a habit. The first is to make a decision to change. When you make a decision, you are committing that you are willing to go to any lengths to make your wishes come true. This means that you will need to completely eliminate the word 'try' from your vocabulary. When you say "I'll try to do my exercises," you are leaving an open door to not doing them. Then in your mind, if you don't do your exercises, that's okay because you only said you would "try" to do them. If you want to successfully change your habits to live a healthier life, you cannot leave an open door to your old habits. You need to just do it, just make the decision and don't look back.

The second thing is to act "as if." Whenever you change what you are doing, it will feel unnatural. It may feel like you are doing something wrong, funny, or something that is just not you. In a way you are right. When you change a habit, you are by definition acting in a way that is 'just not you.' But in a very short time, it will feel normal and it will seem strange that you ever acted any different. Changing habits is like starting a new job, the first couple of weeks are stressful and disorienting, but if you just hang in there, you will feel at home before you know it.

The third and hardest thing that is important to do when you change your bad habits is to get used to feeling a bit uncomfortable. The mind is a very powerful justifier. It tells you over and over again why you are justified in thinking and acting in a certain way. If you decide to quit eating so much sugar, it will take a while before your mind gets used to that idea. In the mean time, you may experience thoughts like "oh, don't make such a big deal out of not eating so much sugar, everybody else eats it," or "who are you kidding, you have always eaten a lot of sugar, that's just who you are." When you hear messages like this bubbling up into your consciousness, just remember that you cannot believe everything you think. As your habits change and you become healthier, your thinking will change right along with it.

A Vision for You

In conclusion, I would just like to encourage you to take your health very seriously. As the old saying goes, if you don't have your health, you don't have anything. Unfortunately, too many people don't discover how true that statement is until it is too late. By simply spending a small amount of your time and energy each day to take care of the most important asset you have - your health - you can improve your quality and length of your life and feel more relaxed and energized.

If you are one of the millions of Americans out there that suffer from neck or back pain, headaches, fibromyalgia, or any other type of pain, you don't have to continue to suffer. You can live without pain through chiropractic care and modest lifestyle changes.

The Healthy Lifestyle Questionnaire

The Healthy Lifestyle Questionnaire is a quick and easy way to gauge the overall healthiness of your current lifestyle habits. Next to each statement or question, simply mark the box which most accurately describes you. Once you have finished answering all the questions, you can score your questionnaire by adding up the numbers in the boxes for each of the statements you checked and plotting them on the chart at the end of this section. You can then use this information to look at ways to change some of your unhealthy habits to healthier ones.

General Health

How do you rate your own Health?	① Above average ③ About average ⑤ Below average
How often do you visit the dentist?	① More than once a year ③ About once a year ⑤ Less than once a year
How often do you visit the Chiropractor?	① At least once evey six weeks ③ Only when I need it ⑤ Rarely or never
What is your cholesterol level?	① Below 210 ③ Above 210 ⑤ Never had it checked
How stressful is your day to day life?	① Very low stress ③ Occasionally stressful ⑤ Very stressful
Are you overweight or under-weight?	① No ③ Yes, by less than 20 pounds ⑤ Yes, by more than 20 pounds

Nutrition

How often do you take a multivitamin?	① Every day ③ Occasionally ⑤ Rarely or never
How often do you consume fast food?	① Less than once a week ③ About once or twice a week ⑤ More than twice a week
How many servings of fruits and vegetables do you consume each day?	① More than five servings ③ Three to five servings ⑤ Fewer than three servings
How much pure water do you drink each day?	① More than 64 oz. ③ Between 32 oz. and 64 oz. ⑤ Less than 32 oz.
How many servings of sweets do you consume each day, such as ice cream, candy, cookies, donuts, etc.?	① Less than one ③ Between one and three ⑤ More than three
How often do you eat a high-protein breakfast?	① Every day ③ At least once per week ⑤ Rarely or never

Recreation and Activity

Overall, how physically active are you?	① Very athletic ③ Moderately physically active ⑤ Mildly physically active
How physically demanding is your job?	① Moderately demanding ③ Very physically demanding ⑤ Not very demanding
How many hours per week do you spend doing vigorous exercise?	① More than four hours ③ Two to four hours ⑤ Fewer than two hours
How often do you stretch your muscles?	① Daily ③ Occasionally ⑤ Rarely or never
How often do you participate in recreational sports, such as golf, swimming, tennis, etc.?	① At least once a week ③ About once per month ⑤ Less than once per month
How many miles per week do you run, jog, or briskly walk?	① More than five miles ③ One to five miles ⑤ Less than one mile

Other Habits

How often do you use tobacco?	① Rarely or never ③ Less than once per week ⑤ At least once per week
How much alcohol do you consume?	① None or very little ③ Less than one drink per day ⑤ More than one drink per day
How often do you use recreational drugs, such as marijuana, amphetamines or cocaine?	① Never ③ Less than once per month ⑤ At least once per month
How many hours of restful sleep do you get each night?	① Six to eight hours ③ More than nine hours ⑤ Five hours or fewer
How is your relationship with the person closest to you?	① Excellent ③ Occasionally problematic ⑤ Frequently troubled
How satisfied are you with your life right now?	① Satisfied ③ Somewhat satisfied ⑤ Unsatisfied

Turn to the next page to score your questionnaire.

Scoring Your Questionnaire

There is a number inside the square next to each answer you checked. Add up the total for each section and enter them below. Add these numbers together to get your total score.

General Health: ______________
Nutrition: ______________
Recreation and Activity: ______________
Other Habits: ______________
Total: ______________

Interpreting Your Score:

101-125 - Poor Lifestyle Habits. You are at a high risk for developing preventible health conditions.

76-100 - Borderline Lifestyle Habits. You have a moderately high risk for developing preventible health conditions.

51-75 - Good Lifestyle Habits. You have a moderately low risk for developing preventible health conditions.

25-50 - Excellent Lifestyle Habits. You have a very low risk of developing preventible health conditions.

About Dr. Stephanie Maj

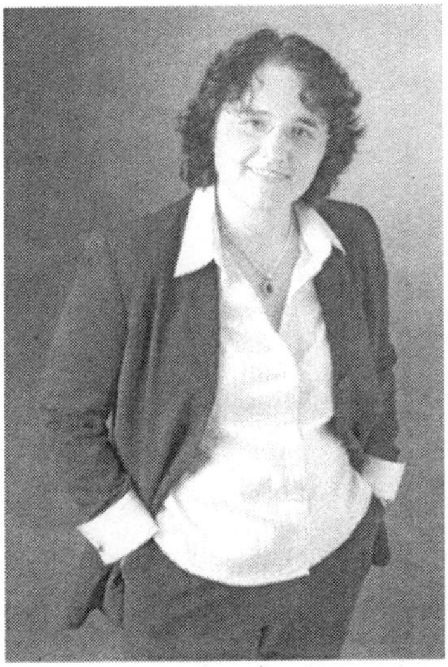

Dr. Stephanie Maj earned her Bachelor of Science in Clinical Nutrition from Ohio University in 1988 and her Doctor of Chiropractic from National College of Chiropractic in 1994. Since 1996, Dr. Maj has owned a family-oriented wellness practice in the Chicago area where she specializes in pregnancy, pediatric, family, and wellness care.

Dr. Maj is certified in Pediatrics from the International Chiropractic Pediatric Association where she completed over 120 hours of curriculum, offering techniques and protocols of care for children and pregnant women. She also earned a Certificate of Proficiency in the Webster Technique, a specific analysis and adjustment used for pregnant women.

Dr. Maj is a member of the International Chiropractic Pediatric Association, the World Chiropractic Alliance-Council on Women's Health, the Chiropractic Leadership Alliance, the National Wellness Foundation, Illinois Prairie State Chiropractic Association, and the International Chiropractic Association. She currently lives in Chicago were she is in private practice.

To Order Copies of This Book

To order additional copies of this book,
please contact my office at:

Community Chiropractic
1442 West Belmont Avenue
Suite 1 East Chicago,IL 60657
(773) 528-8485

Or visity my web site at:
www.YouCanBeWell.net

CPSIA information can be obtained at www.ICGtesting.com
Printed in the USA
LVOW10s0812230114

370641LV00003B/3/P

9 781933 889399